AN EVOLUTION
OF EMPOWERMENT

AN EVOLUTION OF EMPOWERMENT

Voices of Women in Medicine and Their Allies

Shikha Jain, MD

Avital Y. O'Glasser, MD

gatekeeper press™
Tampa, Florida

AN EVOLUTION OF EMPOWERMENT:
Voices of Women in Medicine and Their Allies

Published by Gatekeeper Press
7853 Gunn Hwy., Suite 209
Tampa, FL 33626
www.GatekeeperPress.com

Library of Congress Control Number: 2023943847

ISBN (paperback): 9781662942082
eISBN: 9781662942099

Cover Art by Davy Ran, MD, MSc, MPH

DEDICATION

**To our ancestors, mentors, sponsors, allies,
and those who came before us.**

We stand on the shoulders of giants.

Editors' Introduction

Dr. Shikha Jain and Dr. Avital O'Glasser

Change is happening.

In order for real change to continue, it is imperative that all of us—regardless of gender, status, or position—speak up and work toward change and growth. Too often, the voices of those who need to be heard the most urgently are the ones that are silenced. If we do not speak up, history has repeatedly shown, the inequities will persist. The "we" referred to are those of us who exist in our gender-marginalized communities and populations. We live in societies that are taking three steps forward and twenty steps back. Because of this regression, we need more empowered voices to defend those forward steps and to drive more progress against those twenty steps back as evidenced when policies that were intended to encourage and work toward equity by addressing systemic racism and sexism are rolled back. Women face inequities in our lives—outward microaggressions with comments on pregnancy or our appearance or our intelligence questioned—that erase our voices and discount our opinions. Each of us have existed in the space where, in order to be heard, we need to make sure we are not seen as: too opinionated, too loud, too angry, too bubbly, too bossy, too much. We rely on allies to amplify our voices, lest we are labeled the "b-word" or worse. We have been bullied, gaslighted, sexually harrassed, overlooked, and ignored. And for those with intersectional identities, the weighty burden amplifies. Yet we persist.

Gender inequities in healthcare have existed since Hippocrates postulated that diseases had natural, rather than supernatural, causes. Stereotypes and gender imbalance are woven into the makeup of our society, and healthcare is no exception. The impact of how these disparities impact our patients is a direct reflection on how these inequities impact our healthcare workers. Data consistently shows that when the people treating the patients are representative of that population, outcomes are better. To this day, we have yet to figure out how to translate this data into real-world solutions that effectively close the gender gap among our workforce; consequently, our ability to close the gender gap in our delivery of care remains a pervasive issue.

The concepts of a leaky healthcare pipeline, structural misogyny, gaslighting, bullying, sexism, racism are not new. While the words we use to describe the same inequities time and time again have evolved, the solutions and strategies to address them, unfortunately, have not caught up. Because we continue to document the data, to share our anecdotes, and to build networks of support, the dialogue is changing. The focus and attention have shifted to identify these inequities as they occur, and to reflect on how to make strategic improvements. It is less taboo to share these stories and call out the bad actors. Yet—while we measure the gaps and make strides here and there, while we articulate the challenges and advocate for our needs, while we commiserate and create community through commonality, and while we delight in our diversity and determination—the work isn't complete, not even close. It often feels like we are barely making a dent.

Change *is* happening. Our loud voices resonate with deep reverberation into our bones, hearts, and souls, and they create even deeper impact as they are amplified and recognized by allies, mentors, sponsors, and ourselves. We are at a watershed moment in our history, and the time is now to lift up the voices of those who need to be heard as we strive for greater change at greater speed.

In July 2021, just over a year into the global COVID-19 pandemic, Women in Medicine™ and the Women in Medicine Summit (WIMS) put out a call for original work about gender inequity in healthcare. We could not have anticipated how many people— female, non-binary individuals, and male allies—would trust us to share their words and their work through our platform. Inspired by our authors, we curated this anthology as a symphony of amazing, empowered voices. As you will see, their voices are powerful in their plethora and diversity, as thematic arcs emerge and pull you deeper into their messages. These authors speak to the need for ongoing gender equity and empowerment of women—AND they speak to the incredible and impactful equity advocacy women are accomplishing beyond their specific gendered space WHEN women are empowered. We thank you for honoring them as you read.

Invited Preface

Kimberly Manning, MD

Who do you think you are?

A woman enters a professional space traditionally inhabited by men. Her shoulders are squared, and her expression is determined. As she steps over the threshold, her eyes are trained straight ahead, determinedly landing on each person in her path. With a smile and a nod, she positions herself in the front of the room as the leader. That's when the question splashes her across the cheek like an open hand.

Who do you think you are?

It comes as a whisper. Nearly inaudible at first, but she can hear it. This grating query that challenges her belonging and the audacity with which she entered that room. She clears her throat and tries to ignore it. Finally, she begins to speak, careful to engage her diaphragm and lift her voice to increase her psychological size. From the corner of her eye, she notices two people staring at smartphones as she speaks. Another raises a hand within moments of her beginning to talk. Three others begin a quiet conversation at the back of the room that continues longer than is comfortable or respectful. The tiny voice begs that question again—this time even louder.

Who do you think you are?

....

She finishes her talk points and takes a few questions. Some are rhetorical questions meant only to serve as preambles to self-aggrandizing commentary. The murmurs of those conversing at the end of the table rise slightly above that of comfortable ambient noise and now even more necks curve unapologetically toward texting thumbs on laps. She shifts on her feet and releases a plume of defeated air from her chest. The little voice is now laced with a sarcastic chuckle.

Who do you think you are?

....

She freezes in place. Everyone seems to move in slow motion, and she feels herself shrinking. And just before she nearly disappears, something catches her eye. Or rather, someone. Another woman—one several years her junior. Her face alight, her chin perched up, and her body facing the front of the room. The young woman is at rapt attention, enamored by this speaker who reflects her aspirations. She is taking it all in. Her head dips only to track the notes she has feverishly written in a notebook before her, then darts back upward.

Who do you think you are?

In that moment, the woman at the front of the room feels herself reinflating. The fear and angst she felt moments before is replaced with a mission-driven tenacity to own her space. Now it isn't just her space—it's *their* space. She steps around the table and begins to walk near her seated colleagues. A question is posed to the room that is initially met with silence. She repeats it, this time louder. Someone offers a response, and she probes further. Others chime in and eventually, a robust discussion ensues. She feels herself regaining control, drawing others in, and creating a climate of collaboration. As the conversation begins to subside, she pauses and turns to the young woman in the back—her searing eye contact inviting her to contribute her thoughts. And she does.

Who do you think you are?

This time she said it out loud. It dawns on her that the most important answer to that question begins and ends with her. She recognizes that she can gather strength from her kindred, inspiration from her predecessors, and motivation from those coming behind her. Who she thinks she is and who she believes she can be is intertwined with them.

Who do you think you are?

The years go by, and she grows older and more experienced. The silver streaks at her temples and the crow's feet bursting from her eyes like sunbeams command more respect when she enters a room. And perhaps, with time, the culture has evolved as well. But inside, she still remembers that tiny voice that chastised her all those years before and that lone little sister who counted on her to ignore it.

Who do you think you are?

No, she says. The better question is—who do you *know* you are? And the answer she knows now is the one she wished she'd known back then:

I am enough.

The anthology of voices assembled in this book represents many of us. It is the woman who stood before that room, the little sister who watched with locked eyes from the back, and countless others whose experiences vary as widely as their identities. In medicine and beyond, we recognize that we are stronger together— empowering one another through our stories, deeds, examples, and presence. May these words launch your feet into the heavens to soar and, when you do, may your wings carry others with you. Because we are strong as individuals but even stronger together.

Table of Contents

SECTION ONE

1

"Us"

Any discussion about being a woman in medicine—the joys, thrills, benefits, and the challenges—begins with us articulating and honoring our identities. Our experiences are both universal and individual. We start this anthology with pieces that epitomize how we bear witness and how powerful—and necessary—our testimony must be (Chapter 1). We bear witness to our challenges and successes, especially in the many roles we carry (Chapter 2). However, because bearing witness and carrying multiple roles is exhausting and often demoralizing, we will then read about burnout, imposter syndrome, and wellness (Chapter 3). Finally, the first-person single voice will transcend to the first-person plural voice as we explore the theme of community (Chapter 4).

Chapter 1

BEARING WITNESS

Call Me Cassandra

Avital O'Glasser, MD, FACP, SFHM, DFPM

Eighteen months into the COVID-19 pandemic, I have felt like a Cassandra more and more frequently.

I have a soft spot for Greek mythology, and the less well-known character Cassandra has resonated with me for years. Who was she?

According to the myths, Cassandra, a daughter of King Priam and Queen Hecuba, was a Trojan priestess of Apollo who was cursed to utter true prophecies but to never be believed. Her resulting treatment was awful and dehumanizing: depending on the telling of the myth, she is viewed as a liar, an idiot, or mentally ill.

Just as we can thank Greek mythology for the Oedipus complex, we also have the Cassandra complex. As the centuries have progressed, "Cassandra" metaphorically or rhetorically began to refer to someone whose valid (and ultimately accurate) predictions and warnings are not believed and indeed outright dismissed. Between the 1960s and 1980s, several psychologists, including Laurie Layton Schapira, described the Cassandra complex as a state when women are disbelieved and labeled as histrionic when attempting to share their perspective on emotional or physical suffering.[1] The term has been applied to politics, climate change, and economics. You see where I'm going with this one, right?

There have been multiple Cassandra references in popular culture in recent decades. In the 1995 film *Mighty Aphrodite*, actor Danielle Ferland has a small role as Cassandra, delivering the lines "I see disaster. I see catastrophe" to the assembled Greek chorus.[2] In the powerful novel about the women of the Trojan War, *A Thousand Ships*,[3] Cassandra is viewed by her family as a blubbering, incomprehensible fool—but treated compassionately by the author because of the pain she experiences from the prophecies she receives and because she is never believed.

Since the onset of the COVID-19 era, healthcare professionals have been warning, pleading with, and begging the public to take heed. We've gone from being called heroes, to being ignored, to being yelled and screamed at for continuing to advocate for masks, vaccines, and physical distancing. Many have been on the receiving end of vitriol from sick and dying patients who refuse to accept or believe that they themselves have COVID. Our moral injury is our Cassandra complex.

We are Cassandras.

"I've felt like a Cassandra for months."[4]

---

1 Schapira, Laurie Layton (1988). *The Cassandra Complex: Living With Disbelief: a Modern Perspective on Hysteria* Toronto, Canada: Inner City Books.

2 *Mighty Aphrodite.* Directed by Woody Allen, Miramax, 1996.

3 Haynes, Natalie. *A Thousand Ships: A Novel.* Harper, an Imprint of HarperCollins Limited, 2021.

4 Avital Y. O'Glasser, MD FACP SFHM DFPM [@aoglasser]. "And the Pandemic Is Still Going on It's Bad. It's Really Bad. My Overwhelming Emotion Right Now Is Anger. Yes There's a Lot of Fear and Anxiety-but Anger. and Exhaustion-Mental, Physical, Emotional. I've Felt like a Cassandra for Months (Don't Know the Reference? Look It up)." Twitter, 7 Aug. 2021, https://twitter.com/aoglasser/status/1424075305304563717?s=20.

"But I'm a Cassandra."[5]

"'Just call me Cassandra,' every frontline COVID provider and public health official."[6]

"Cursed with the gift of "'I told you so' and 'gosh you were rights'..."[7]

According to the myths, Cassandra is ultimately deemed worthy of her dedication. To my fellow sister Cassandras—I HEAR you. I SEE you. I BELIEVE you. I know others do as well. Keep advocating and warning. We are not cursed to never be believed.

---

5 Jane van Dis MD. [@janevandis]. "I Actually Feel Guilty as the OBGYN for Flashes When I'm Delivering a Newborn. but I'm a Cassandra." Twitter, 3 Apr. 2021, https://twitter.com/janevandis/status/1378484140002058242?s=20.

6 Gretchen Diemer [@gretchendiemer]. "'Just Call Me Cassandra," Every Frontline Covid Provider and Public Health Official. #COVID19 Pic.twitter.com/su2rFBKGbb." Twitter, 26 July 2021, https://twitter.com/gretchendiemer/status/1419468199364546560?s=20.

7 Midwest Prole [@midwestprole]. "Same Cassandra Feeling—cursed with the Gift of 'I Told You so' and 'Gosh You Were Rights' . . . Anyone without Blinders on Can See That We Are about to Sacrifice Our Children on the Altar of Baal (Politics / Capitalism / Ego Cults).It's Going to Take Pediatric Deaths?! JFC! Https://T.co/e3koborgc8." Twitter, 9 Aug. 2021, https://twitter.com/MidwestProle/status/1424530432104742914?s=20.

Serious Hair

Jennifer Lycette, MD

If you want to be taken seriously, you have to have serious hair.

That line has lived in my brain since 1988. I was fifteen years old, and I was convinced Melanie Griffith's character in *Working Girl* had revealed one of life's secret truths. In the movie, she utters the line as she directs her friend to lop off her long blonde mane. All so her new boss, played by Sigourney Weaver, will take her seriously in the workplace.

As a teenager in the '80s, it was obvious as I looked ahead to college and "escaping" my hometown that this was the secret to success I'd been searching for. After all, could Sigourney Weaver have fought off the Alien if she hadn't had serious hair?

No doubt, much of my fascination with the potential of what a radical haircut could hold for a woman came from the fact that my father had forbidden short hair. So, it will come as little surprise to the reader here to learn that shortly after I "escaped" to college, I took myself to a salon.

"Cut it short," I declared.

The stylist raised an eyebrow but made quick work of it. For the first time, my hair ended above my shoulders. I reveled in my new style. I felt older, freer, lighter.

But did people take me more seriously? A hometown friend commented when I returned for winter break, "You look like someone from *90210*." (Note to Gen Z: this was considered a compliment in the early '90s). Still, not exactly the vibe I'd been going for.

The lessons from the movies of my coming-of-age years continued. In 1995, *Legends of the Fall* came out. I recall being home on college break and watching it with my family. Afterward, my dad turned to me with a perplexed expression. "But why did she cut off her hair?" He was referring to Julia Ormond's character.

I struggled to find the words to reply. Was he asking about the movie? Or something more. A multitude of thoughts went through my mind. *To be free. To express herself. To be her own person. To take control. To leave bad memories behind.*

What I said out loud—with a falsely nonchalant shrug—was this: "I don't know."

A few years later, toward the end of my time at medical school, my then-boyfriend (now-husband) and I set a wedding date, and without discussion, I let my hair grow out long again. He didn't care about my hair length, but it would seem I couldn't get past the social conditioning of my childhood—a bride "needed" long hair.

But in residency, when I decided to apply to Hematology/Oncology fellowship, I cut it short again. I couldn't envision how I'd tell my patients the treatments I'd be recommending would cause hair loss if I was sitting in front of them with long hair myself. Besides that, I thought it would also head off the constant comment: "You don't look old enough to be a doctor."

But no matter my hair length, those comments persisted. For the years that followed, I continued striving to find the ultimate style for "serious hair" that would garner respect in the workplace. But I could never seem to get it quite right. I tried them all—the classic bob, the long pixie, the angled bob, the lob. But no matter the style, I could still be asked at the end of a patient interaction, "When do I get to see the doctor?"

At the same time, I want to acknowledge the privilege I've had as a white woman physician. Women of color suffer from even more macro and microaggressions over the appearance of hair. In a 2020 *New York Times* interview, Dr. Onyeka Otugo, an emergency medicine attending physician and health policy fellow at Brigham and Women's Hospital, shared how many medical students feared negative repercussions to their grades and performance evaluations if they wore their hair naturally.[8]

As the years went on, no matter my hair length, the questions and comments persisted—even two decades after medical school—mostly from patients, but also colleagues. Recently when starting a new job fifteen years post-fellowship, a male physician who didn't know me (or my CV) repeatedly suggested I "run my cases by" another colleague, as if I was a trainee. My hair still wasn't serious enough. And apparently, I was ageless. Unless the problem was never my appearance—but my femaleness.

So, when the pandemic came, and I stopped going to the salon, I welcomed the relaxation of society's "style rules" for women. My hair grew. I didn't pay attention to it. Pulling it into a quick ponytail for work took all of thirty seconds. For the first time since adoles-

---

8 Goldberg, Emma. "For Doctors of Color, Microaggressions Are All Too Familiar." *The New York Times*, 11 Aug. 2020, https://www.nytimes.com/2020/08/11/health/microaggression-medicine-doctors.html.

cence, I didn't care what anyone thought of my hair. We were in a pandemic, people.

Then, I attended my first, small, in-person work meeting (masked and socially distanced, of course). The biggest surprise wasn't how awkward it felt to be with people outside my department for the first time in over a year. It was the hairstyles of the other women. Salon-quality cuts and color. All different lengths. I couldn't stop gaping. It felt like a betrayal—I thought we had an agreement.

So one day, I gave in and booked an appointment online (I'm fully vaccinated, and the salon requires masks). It's been over 18 months since my last salon haircut. Will I emerge from the salon with serious hair?

No matter the length of my hair, the answer is no. Because like so many expectations society puts on women, the pandemic has helped me see such a thing doesn't exist.

Sorry, Melanie.

Unwomen

Kristina Domanski, MD

In Margaret Atwood's *The Handmaid's Tale,*[9] a woman can be an Unwoman, a Martha, or a Handmaid. "Unwomen" are the sterile women, the women not married to a man, lesbian and bisexual women, vocal and politically dissident women: women who are incapable of integration within Gilead's strict gender roles. The House of Medicine, in particular academic medicine, is its own Gilead. Women have a clearly defined set of roles as well as a set of rules, behavioral and clothing standards that apply only to them. Both the roles and the rules were dreamed up by men. Anyone who does not comply is an Unwoman.

Marthas do the grunt work in academic medicine, churning out research papers that men's names get attached to, participating in committees chaired by men, setting up venues and catering for Residency events that the male faculty just show up to. Despite their productivity, Marthas are not respected or appropriately financially compensated. The gender pay gap still exists. Most importantly, Marthas are not promoted and the leadership pipeline continues to hemorrhage women.

---

9 Atwood, Margaret. *The Handmaid's Tale.* New York: Everyday Library, 2006.

Our female residents are Handmaids, owned and controlled by the House. The average Handmaid has hundreds of thousands of dollars of debt and must endure whatever abuse is thrown at her in order to pay it. While we are miles away from the atrocious work hours of the 1980s, residency is hard work coupled with emotional labor. Handmaids navigate a minefield that can vary from frankly egregious sexual harassment, to more subtle microaggressions that happen in plain sight and are so ingrained in residency culture that they become routinely accepted. A Handmaid who speaks up is promptly muzzled, branded, or otherwise scarred. We carry those scars out of residency and into our professional careers.

And then there are Unwomen. They are the women who dare to question the status quo, who speak up when they are interrupted or talked over, who refuse to start every sentence with "I'm sorry" or "Is it ok if . . .", who make no apologies for their voices or their femininity. They are the women whose situation prevents them from speaking publicly, but who do important work on the inside. These women are reading articles such as Dr. Erica Kaye's[10] and getting angry that a profession built on the foundation of "do no harm" is rotten to the core and riddled with systemic sexism.

Gilead exiles Unwomen to "the Colonies," areas both of agricultural production and of radioactive pollution. Medicine exiles us to a peculiar limbo where we are viewed with suspicion by the majority of men, as well as some of the women who choose to follow the rules. Our lifespan is uncertain. We are allowed to stay in the Colonies as long as we are able to reach the required level of clinical and academic productivity. Our work is made more difficult than that of a Martha, and we do it in a toxic environment in which our

10 Kaye EC. Misogyny in Medicine. N Engl J Med. 2021 Jun 17;384(24):2267-2269.

physical and mental health slowly declines. We are painfully aware that even if we don't succumb to the unacceptably high levels of radiation, we are always just a few steps away from being sent to the Wall for capital punishment.

The Wall is reserved for those of us deemed resistant to correctional therapy in the form of "Professionalism" seminars, HR write-ups, and mansplaining about how we should be "more approachable" and "less intimidating." Anyone who dares to call out the behavioral double standard, verbally or in writing, gets sent to the Wall. Question a high-up Commander's leadership style? Yup, the Wall. Once we are hung from the Wall, we get labeled "troublemakers" and put on lists that deem us unhireable. We are railroaded out of academia and our voices silenced with the chilling and swift effectiveness of a noose around the neck.

As I meet another new class of interns, I wonder not only how many future Unwomen I am welcoming into the Colonies, but how to prepare them for the path ahead. I also wonder whether I am doing them a disservice by teaching them to speak up and call out the microaggressions, the double standards, and all the other sexist delights the House of Medicine has to offer. I have been thinking about this question for some time, and the best answer I can come up with is to be transparent. I will never lead someone blindfolded into the Colonies, but will welcome with open arms anyone who enters willingly. The more of us there are, the louder our collective voice. And realistically, they can't send all of us to the Wall.

Galadriel, Girl, You're Being Gaslit

Jennifer Lycette, MD

Galadriel, you may be the Elf Commander of the Northern Armies, the Warrior of the Wastelands, and the Lady of the woods of Lothlórien, but I am a human woman and, therefore, in a unique position to teach you something (perhaps the only thing) mortal women know better than Elven women: gaslighting.

What is this gaslighting I speak of? No, it's not a light for dark places when all other lights go out. Ever hear of Cassandra? (Oh, wait, never mind, wrong mythology. But you would like her.) Gaslighting is the psychological manipulation of someone for the purpose of making them call into question their own sanity—something human men have done to women in my world for millennia.

I fear your pals Elrond and King Gil-Galad have been hanging around the men of Middle-Earth and absorbing some of their least savory characteristics. You say they don't deign to the company of mortal men? I counter, where else could they have learned the soul-destroying machinations of gaslighting? The dwarves? I think not. Have you ever seen a dwarven woman put up with a word of male nonsense? I rest my case.

You still doubt me, I see. Let me ask you this. After your soldiers mutinied against you and you returned to Lindon, what did King Gil-Gilad do? Did he listen to your explanation of your findings of the ongoing evil in Middle-Earth? Or provide you any sort of support to continue your mission? Not to mention, reprimand your soldiers for questioning your lifetime of expertise (and by lifetime, of course, I mean eons) and disobeying your orders?

No. Gil-Gilad dismissed your concerns and your evidence. He ignored your lived experience and told you the war was over, despite your firsthand proof to the contrary. You, the *Commander of the Northern Armies.* He literally tried to *ship you off.*

"You've been working so hard, Galadriel," he said. "Take a vacation. Don't worry your pretty little head about any of this. Go to Valinor. Have some 'you' time. You deserve it." (I paraphrase, of course.)

But we all know what he really meant was, *"We don't need your relentless pursuit of the truth and your inconvenient questions, which make me look bad, and really, you're costing us so much in terms of resources, can't you just look the other way and pretend it's all good?"*

And your friend, Elrond, what did he do? Did he step up to have your back? No. He, in his youthful folly, presumed to know what was best for you (even if he *knew* it wasn't exactly the truth) and supported Gil-Galad. This is an essential component of human gaslighting. The group (those in power, often men) conspires against the individual (usually someone questioning the power structure, often a woman).

At this point, you weren't sure what was happening. I saw your confusion. Your frustration that you weren't being heard. Why was no one listening to you? You're the *Commander of the Northern Armies.* Why were they ignoring the evidence you brought to them?

When they manipulated you to step onto that boat to Valinor, you wondered if you were going crazy, right? A-ha! That's gaslighting.

Thankfully for the rest of Middle-Earth, you knew to trust yourself best and dove into the icy waters of truth just in time.

It will be cold comfort indeed when I tell you that shortly after his failed attempt to ship you off, King Gil-Gilad discovered the rot in the trees of Lindor was still spreading. Imagine that. Getting rid of the pesky female messenger *didn't* eliminate the deep-rooted disaster of which you were only trying to warn him.

But any woman could have told him that.

Ask Cassandra.

May Her Memory Be a Revolution

Avital O'Glasser, MD, FACP, SFHM, DFPM

Do you remember where you were or what you were doing in 2020 when you learned that Ruth Bader Ginsberg had passed away? I do.

I had just gone outside after it had rained—the first substantial rain we received after a horrific stretch of Oregon wildfires during the horrific first six months of the pandemic. I was standing outside, breathing in clean air for the first time in two weeks, and I tweeted that "it really felt like the physical and metaphysical 'separation' I needed" going into the new year.[11] It really felt like a demarcation, and with it brought a new hope that the evil, pain, and sadness of the preceding year would be washed away. It was quite literally a new breath of air and a new hope for the coming year.

And then it all came crashing down during Rosh Hashanah (sundown on September 18th). Rosh Hashanah is one of the holiest

---

11 Avital Y. O'Glasser, MD FACP SFHM DFPM (she/her) [@aoglasser]. "I Hope so!It Really Felt like the Physical and Metaphysical 'Separation' I Needed Mentally between 5780 and 5781." Twitter, 18 Sept. 2020, https://twitter.com/aoglasser/status/1307018118120628224?s=20&t=0S07dwLXvBlLuGkfPR7dDg.

days of the Jewish year in addition to Yom Kippur. For Rosh Hashanah, we wish people a "sweet new year," sweet like the honey we dip apples in. May our "sweet" year be sweet in connection, sweet in engagement, sweet in deeply meaningful acts and experiences, and sweet in being constructive rather than destructive. Shortly after the start of Rosh Hashanah on the East Coast, and shortly before the start of Rosh Hashanah where I lived on the West Coast, all the hope and joy and optimism was ripped out from under us. We learned that RBG had died.

The fall Jewish High Holidays focus their imagery and spiritual weight on being evaluated for your past year. We reference the Book of Life and the Book of Death. Strictest interpretations and traditions believe that our fate for the coming year—life or death— is decided that week. There are many modernistic interpretations of this that are less fatalistic and instead focus on "how" we live, not "if" we live.

But Jewish tradition also has a very interesting interpretation of what it means to die at that transition point of the year—that these are the most righteous people amongst us. Nina Totenberg shared this wisdom the night of RBG's death: "A Jewish teaching says that those who die just before the Jewish new year are the ones that God has held back until the last moment because they were needed most and were the most righteous."[12] Even though one is destined to die in a specific calendar year, God holds back until the very last moment in order for someone to maximize the

12 Nina Totenberg [@NinaTotenberg]. "A Jewish Teaching Says Those Who Die Just before the Jewish New Year Are the Ones God Has Held Back until the Last Moment BC They Were Needed Most & Were the Most Righteous. and so It Was That #RBG Died as the Sun Was Setting Last Night Marking the Beginning of Roshhashanah." Twitter, 19 Sept. 2020, https://twitter.com/NinaTotenberg/status/1307169055313457152?s=20&t=mcxo1fsDEqOA51BVssrmKg.

good they brought to the world. My own grandmother died the night before Rosh Hashanah fourteen years ago. So, the significance of the timing was not new to me in 2020 as my family turned to that ancient belief as some small source of comfort in our mourning. That powerful ancient tradition brought a new gravitas to RBG's death that holiday period.

Part of the Yom Kippur service involves beating our breasts as a sign of atonement—and we did that a week after RBG's death. But many women and allies—Jewish and non-Jewish—beat our breasts during that Rosh Hashanah as we feared what was to come with the open Supreme Court seat during the Trump presidency. The emotions and the fear, especially for the fate of women and other vulnerable members of our society, were real and raw.

And two years later, we were sadly validated. Those who gaslighted us and told us not to be histrionic have been proven wrong. Our Cassandras have been proven correct. Our anticipatory sorrow has since materialized in many ways, including the June 2022 decision in the Dobbs case that overturned *Roe v. Wade* and—mirroring our sorrow two years earlier—the descending apparition carried the power refrain "With Sorrow."[13]

On the anniversary of a loved one's death, Jews say the Mourners' Kaddish, the Mourner's Prayer. But mourning, and remembering one's passing even years later, is not about being locked in the past. It's about looking forward. It's about memory and legacy. Jews do not say "rest in peace." We say *zichron l'bracha*–"may her memory be a blessing."

"May her memory be a BLESSING." This may be ringing a bell.

13 Dobbs v. Jackson Women's Health Organization, 597 U. S. ___ (2022)

"May her memory be a REVOLUTION!" You may have seen that rallying cry years ago. For many, RBG's death and the timing of her death were a call that "we all need to work for justice."[14]

It was a long two years, a very long two years. The dangers in the world that we need to fight against persist—from COVID-19 to attacks on abortion access to gun violence to climate change, from structural racism to misogyny to the "phobias" (transphobia, homophobia, xenophobia, and more). Politicians continue to use the legal and political system to perpetuate these dangerously hateful attitudes—and the courts stacked by the former president continue to contribute to this. But this is not without opposition. Many, especially women, continue to work to live up to RBG's edict that women "belong in all the places where decisions are being made."[15]

There is work to be done. So, let's do it!

There is activism and advocacy to be done. So, let us do it!

RBG's closest family will stand up again and recite the Mourner's Prayer. At the Yom Kippur service next week, many will attend the traditional annual memorial service. We will pray that the memories we remember will be blessings and fuel. May RBG's memory continue to be a blessing; may it continue to be a revolution!

---

14 Ruttenberg, Danya. "Perspective | Jewish Tradition Calls on the Rest of Us to Act in Ginsburg's Memory." The Washington Post, 22 Sept. 2020, https://www.washingtonpost.com/outlook/2020/09/22/ginsburg-rosh-hashanah-tzaddik/.

15 "Ruth Bader Ginsburg in Pictures and Her Own Words." BBC News, 19 Sept. 2020, https://www.bbc.com/news/world-us-canada-54218139.

Chapter 2

ROLES WE CARRY

A Reminder of Real Love

Mehak Dagar

A medical student with a bag of O negative blood, running eccentrically through the hospital corridor to make sure the blood reaches the OR on time,

A nurse hunching over a patient's chest with all her strength trying to get a pulse,

A surgeon who just identified a bleeder and ligated it,

An obstetric surgeon who delivered a baby stuck by its own head,

An orthopedic surgeon who took that limb away only to see her patient take up a new sport,

An anesthesiologist who got a bilateral air entry on a difficult intubation,

A plastic surgeon whose patient finally loves her new nose,

A psychiatrist who sees her suicidal patient living a healthy life.

And many more such women in medicine.

Each one of them, in their own way, saves a life every day.

Someone stays up the whole night monitoring a patient's urine output,

A mother misses her daughter's first birthday to stitch up a wound,

A daughter turns up at last for a family dinner, late again after attending to someone else's ailing family member.

We lose a lot of things that can never be bought back by money,

There is no "best employee of the month,"

No badges,

No stars,

No one asks for a selfie with that doctor who saved their lives,

No pat on the back.

From managing 300 patients a day to being mocked for missing the mention of one patient's blood pressure, we have seen it all.

It's our job. We chose it. We're assumed to be okay.

Except—

The cardiac monitor showing a pulse after a pulseless electrical activity,

The flat line in the ECG showing a P wave,

That. That is our appraisal, the life we just saved.

And when we realize we have the power to do so, there is nothing more addictive,

Nothing more sickening,

Nothing more maddening than medical science.

Nothing else can give you an adrenaline rush so powerful. We give up our own lives for theirs, but in hindsight, every bit of it is worth it. No one pats our back; we pat our own back,

We are our own protagonist,

We wear our own cape and crown,

We save our own selves and we save them,

This love-hate relationship makes us a Doctor.

We practice real love.

Medicine Is Personal: Deep Down to My Soul

Anuja Dattatray Mali

To know even one life has breathed easier because
you have lived. This is to have succeeded.

—RALPH WALDO EMERSON

One of the truths about choosing to study medicine is that, from the moment you decide to go down that road, you are bombarded with the same question.

Why medicine?

You'd think that once you get into medical school, you'll never be asked that question ever again, but you are.

I am a first-year medical student aspiring to become a surgeon. I know, I know.

SURGERY?

How are you so sure about it?

You have just started your med school.

You haven't even seen the patients.

Do you even know how much time and hard work it takes to become a renowned surgeon?

So, how do I respond when people ask me if I'm scared about how long it takes to become a doctor? There's the classic refrain, *You'll get older anyways, so you may as well be a doctor!"*

For me, this is different. There is a special joy that comes with the practice of surgery. Surgeons, indeed, are distinguished by the art and craft of their ability to perform surgical procedures or operations. And as a disclaimer: the length of training is a non-issue to me. We live our dream every day, and if it's what you want and what you're passionate about, there is no reason to elude your calling.

Each person defines success in different ways. To know that even one life will be improved by my actions affords me immense gratification and meaning. That is success to me. I want to have the ability to provide care and treatment on a daily basis as a physician. I hope to not only care for patients with the same compassion with which physicians do, but to add to the daily impact I can have by tackling large-scale issues in health, and to not forget the days when I'll do my first surgery, when I'll treat my first patient or when I will listen to the heartbeat of the first child I'll deliver as a doctor.

There is something sacred, even empowering, about providing support when people need it the most. I think medicine is rewarding and eye-opening while simultaneously challenging. Helping people at their most vulnerable time is a privilege. To me, empathy is the essence.

My reason for sticking with medicine from sixth grade is due to my intrinsic and fierce desire to help and to save the lives of others. I want to be a hero, not with weapons or superpowers, but with a scalpel. The knight in shining scrubs. It's such a profound feeling that it's quite hard to explain what it's like. It's not something that can be learned; you can't be taught to want to be a doctor.

That intense thirst for medicine, it just *is*, and there is truly no other way to put it.

Truth be told, it's not something you can explain in simple terms. It's a very personal dream, a very strong dream, and the desire to help others is unexplainable. You're the only one who fully knows why you do medicine, and why you want to pursue the hard journey, and why you want to go through it all. I have no doubt that the next ten years will be similarly unpredictable. But I can assure you that no matter what obstacles I face, my goal will remain the same. I know with certainty that this is the profession for me. Medicine is personal, deep down to my soul.

A Brief History of Women in Medicine

Krisa Keute, MD, FACP

A father and son were in a car accident. The father dies and the son is taken to the nearest hospital. In the operating room, a doctor comes in and looks at the little boy and says, "I can't operate on this boy because he is my son." Who is the doctor?

Sometimes I share this riddle with my kids and their friends. More than half of the time they look at me confused and can't figure out the riddle. They scratch their heads and sometimes ask if the surgeon is the stepfather. Could it be the wrong boy in surgery? They look me in the eye, often after a long day of work at the hospital. They forget that I am a doctor, and likely are unaware that by 2021, more women graduated from medical school than men.

Yet, the history of women in medicine began over 150 years ago. The story goes that around about 1844, a young woman lay dying of uterine cancer. She confided in her friend, Elizabeth, that perhaps, had a woman cared for her, she may have been spared suffering and embarrassment. She may have been nurtured through her illness instead of experiencing the sterile, impersonal process she endured at the hands of the men who had cared for her. This honest testament seeded the call to a new vocation for her friend Elizabeth, thus starting a revolution, and shattering a proverbial glass ceiling.

For women physicians, our pioneering hero Elizabeth Blackwell was perhaps the most impressive first of all firsts. She was not only the first woman admitted to medical school, she graduated at the very top of her class (despite discrimination, exclusion from certain lectures deemed "inappropriate" for ladies, and blatant and generally accepted misogyny). She was supremely influential in paving the way for others, including her sister Emily. When most medical schools refused to open their doors to women, she founded her own schools specifically for women. She not only educated women, she remained true to her friend and provided health care to women and children, often indigent, by establishing special infirmaries in the US and Britain specifically for women. Elizabeth Blackwell, who simply listened to her dying friend, not only shattered a glass ceiling, she launched her influence far and wide and soared to great lengths, paving the way for women everywhere to follow in her footsteps.

Time marched forward and subsequently many variations of Elizabeth Blackwells entered medical schools around the globe. Rebecca Lee Crumpler, the first black female doctor (who graduated prior to the end of the Civil War!), Virginia Apgar, champion of newborn health and wellbeing, and Elisabeth Kubler-Ross, expert on death and dying, all achieved an M.D. These are giants in the medical field. When I consider their achievements in the face of discrimination because of gender, my throat tightens with such emotional pride that I want to rejoice—for I get to be a small part of them.

Chapter 2: *Roles We Carry*

Heading to college with the dream of becoming a female physician, I revel in my dream coming true. Interviewing for residency while five months pregnant, I was blatantly asked how I could possibly do it all. I don't think a male parent, obviously not pregnant candidate, got that question. After "somehow" tackling a brutal, at times a hundred-hour work week at Hennepin County Internal Medicine residency, I retained my first job, which included joining eight men, no women, in a pioneering hospitalist program, at age 29. One of my consulting colleagues repeatedly referenced himself as "Dr. So-and-So" while calling me by my first name. He couldn't quite fathom that I was an MD, not a nurse. Yet, years flew by and the practice, the patients, and the colleagues enriched my life beyond any of my wildest expectations. And the best—the very best—part of all of it have been the women I have met along the way.

In the early morning before sunrise, a younger woman physician and I met to run along the north shore of Lake Superior. She—with her youth, her fresh mind, and her idealistic uncertainty about whether she is truly working in a way which fulfills her calling to serve others— and I—with my archaic dog and my twenty years' baggage of being a local with a weary acceptance that I will be a physician forever—begin our sweet, pre-work morning run.

Like many of my female doctor friends, ours is a kindred friendship that often comes naturally with people whose studies, training, and experience mirror one another. It is the kind where two like-minded people find one another and become fast friends. She has about four years' experience under her belt; I have about twenty. She is single with local family; I am a mom of three who is four hours from my nearest kin. She has school loans and an old jalopy Corolla that worries me; I have no more loans and a somewhat unnecessarily sporty Jeep. She is a millennial raised by a bit of a hippie mom; I am a Gen Xer and a latchkey kid. I think this is the start of another beautiful female medical friendship.

We pass the usual morning greetings and start out on the lakewalk, cantering at about the speed of a lazy bat, maybe a sauntering skunk. We talk of our day, some cases, COVID. We banter back and forth about difficulties with patient care, troublesome cases where we are having an arduous time diagnosing or treating disease. We mention colleagues who are giving us trouble and colleagues who are helpful. It is a delight to me, and I revel in having found another female friend to socialize and work with.

The years have given me a loyal, globe-trotting-gynecologist girlfriend, a wine-aficionado-and-foodie-pathologist girlfriend, a med-peds-supermom-of-boys girlfriend who keeps up a sweet long distance relationship with me, among others. It is our own special club, because we are often outsiders in the world of soccer moms, stay-at-home moms, and those others who (thankfully) run the nonmedical logistics of our mom community. We have a special bond, we female physicians.

Women doctors account for one-third of the physicians practicing medicine in America, according to the Kaiser Family Foundation.[16] In 2017, for the first time in history, women entering American medical schools outnumbered men.[17] While exciting to see this transition, according to the 2019 Medscape Physician Compensation Report, the gender pay gap in primary care widened from previous years to a nearly 25% disparity in income, favor-

---

16 Women and Health Care: Key Findings from the Kaiser Women's Health Survey. Kaiser Family Foundation. July 2005.
17 2017 Applicant and Matriculant Data Tables. Association of American Medical Colleges December 2017.

ing men over women.[18] This disparity widened three years after JAMA's bombshell report comparing hospital mortality and readmission rates for 1,583,028 hospitalized Medicare beneficiaries, finding that female physicians had significantly lower mortality rates (adjusted, 11.07% vs 11.49%) and readmission rates (adjusted, 15.02% vs 15.57%) for hospitalized patients.[19] So in essence, female doctors are paid less, but may be giving at least as good, if not better, medical care.

Of course, it really isn't quite as black-and-white as that, and I must be careful not to toot our own female horn too loudly. I remember when that study came out. A few of us women docs were talking about it, and one of our male colleagues (who is a very gifted physician himself) became agitated. Remembering this, I want to point out that while I am proud to be a female doctor, I cannot dismiss that it takes all of us—mentors, colleagues, friends, both male and female—to make our beloved medical practice valuable, successful, compassionate, and altruistic. I believe that we are stronger together, united in our goal of helping women help themselves and help others.

And so I say, "Thank you, Elizabeth Blackwell. Thank you, wonderful female colleagues and friends who enrich my life, my practice. My patients and I are forever indebted to you."

---

18 Medscape Physician Compensation Report 2019. Medscape. Available at: https://www. medscape.com/sites/public/physician-comp/2019

19 Tsugawa Y, Jena AB, Figueroa JF, Orav EJ, Blumenthal DM, Jha AK. Comparison of Hospital Mortality and Readmission Rates for Medicare Patients Treated by Male vs Female Physicians. JAMA Intern Med. 2017;177(2):206–213. doi:10.1001/ jamainternmed.2016.7875

Are Women Surgeons Modern Day Witches?

Sarah M. Temkin, MD

As Halloween approaches, thoughts turn to witches—which means women—but what about the witchiness of those women who are surgeons?

As a woman, a surgeon, and the executive producer of *1001Cuts*, a film designed to explore the barriers to entry and success for women within surgery, I've seen how surgical culture has remained stubbornly inhospitable to women. Passage of the Title IX amendment of the Civil Rights Act in 1972 prohibited discrimination based upon gender by institutions that provide higher education. This paved the way for women to enter medicine. By 1980, thirty percent of medical students in the United States were women, and since 2003, half of students entering medical schools have been women.[20] Yet women continue to be underrepresented in surgery. Only recently has the number of women choosing to train in surgical specialties begun to increase; the percentage of women practicing certain specialties like neurosurgery and or-

---

20 Relman, Arnold S. "Here come the women." *New England Journal of Medicine*, vol. 302, no. 6, May 1980, pp 1252-53. https://www.nejm.org/doi/full/10.1056/nejm198005293022209

thopedic surgery remains in the single digits or in the low double digits.[21]

Surgery is a profession created by and traditionally dominated by men, hence without discursive spaces for women. The environment of the operating room was established to accommodate the prototypical male surgeon. The scrubs fit a male body (no waist). The gloves fit male hands (thick fingers). The handles on surgical instruments are typically too large for an average female hand— some women need to use two hands to use instruments designed to be one-handed. The height of the operating room tables assumes a surgeon height of at least 5 feet 8 inches. Not having equipment or an environment that was made for women is just one part of the messaging received by women in surgery that they do not belong.

Women are expected to be warm and communal, not bold or technically proficient. For simply practicing surgery, making decisions, utilizing equipment correctly, or speaking up about patient safety issues, women are punished for violating gender roles (socially ascribed sets of expectations associated with the perception of masculinity and femininity). Women who are surgeons who have been interviewed for the film describe falling prey to the classic and well-described "double bind."[22] The double bind is the no-win situation women find in the workplace where if they perform well, they'll be perceived as unlikeable, but if they are likable, their competence will be questioned.

---

21 Physician specialty data report. Association of American Medical Colleges.2018. Available at: https://www.aamc.org/data/workforce/reports/492536/2018-physician-specialty-data-report.html

22 IBM Corporation. The Double-Bind Dilemma for Women in Leadership: Damned if You Do, Doomed if You Don't. Catalyst. 2007. https://www.catalyst.org/wp-content/uploads/2019/01/The_Double_Bind_Dilemma_for_Women_in_Leadership_Damned_if_You_Do_Doomed_if_You_Dont.pdf

In many ways, we are still labeled and branded as "witches." Although women are no longer drowned, hung, or burned as witches, many of the roots of our modern social and cultural responses to women holding power (including the power to heal) can be traced to the story of witch. Rounding up and punishing women for violating gender norms and roles was central to the witch hunts of the sixteenth and seventeenth century that swept much of Northern Europe and ultimately reached as far as New England. Although both men and women were accused of witchcraft, women were disproportionately charged and executed for this crime. One of the most common accusations against witches was having the power to affect health—often specifically the possession of midwifery or other medical skills.[23] After being accused, witches underwent a trial by dunking to determine whether they were guilty. If she drowned, she was innocent, if she floated, she had proven herself a witch and was subsequently hung or burned at the stake.

The *"damned if you do, damned if you don't"* outcomes of a witch hunt resonate with many of the stories of surgeons who are women that have been shared in the making of the film. Hardly a surgeon who is a woman has not been called a "word that rhymes with witch [bitch]" at work. The accusations arise from simple acts required to do the job of a surgeon—being assertive, asking for instruments, or staying calm in the face of chaos. Surgeons have described being either too loud or not loud enough, too bubbly or too serious, talking too much or not enough. Efforts to prove that she's a regular surgeon doing her job suddenly become proof that she is indeed a woman in possession of supernatural powers, capable of using dark magic to exercise her will. Broomstick, cauldron, potions, and all

---

23 Ehrenreich, Barbara, and Deirdre English. *Witches, Midwives, and Nurses* (2nd Edition). The Feminist Press, 2010.

are suddenly part of her persona. But sutures, scalpels, and scopes are powerful implements, and with these new tools surgeons who are women can and will make changes to surgical culture. The profession can be transformed and elevated, and patients will benefit.

Motherhood, Medicine, and Equality

Reges A. Hansen, DO

I started medical school with a one-year-old, and I am ending it with three exceptional children under the age of five. We have survived brutal eighty+-hour weeks, a pandemic, a move, a rigorous interview season, MATCH, and a plethora of tantrums (some of them mine). What did this experience teach me? It taught me that although women are generally accepted as equal, competent, and compassionate physicians, something about the role of motherhood negates our "equal-ness."

I think this is best explained by some of the comments that I have received:

Are you hiding your pregnancy from residencies because they will discriminate against you for that?

Who is parenting your children?

Shouldn't you consider nursing so that you can be there for your children?

You have young children, and your husband is already a doctor. Why are you here?

Let me be clear here. Those comments do not deserve a response, but I will answer the last one. I am here as a new psychiatry intern because I believe I will make a difference in the lives of the patients I serve. This will often be the same answer you will hear from my male and female colleagues. However, motherhood has changed me as a person in profound ways. My children have only deepened my compassion and understanding of suffering. It has also exponentially increased my capacity for patience and forgiveness. These are traits essential for work in all fields of medicine.

Motherhood has also brought to light that a phenomenon exists where women own their bodies and careers as long as children are not involved. All of our "equality" is thrown out the window when we are presented with two little lines. Now as we sit on the precipice of women losing fundamental rights over our own bodies, there is continued conversation about who owns pregnancies and motherhood. As a woman who is balancing both a career and motherhood (and only able to do so with the support of my partner and family), there is only one answer: the person who is pregnant is completely responsible for the outcome of those decisions.

The Perpetual "Yes"

Elizabeth Rubin, MD

Yes. Sure. Of course. No problem. I got it. Let me help you. How can I help you? What can I do for you? I'll figure it out. We can work it out. I'll do it. I would love to. Seems great, thanks!

My whole life has been about compliance. People pleasing. Pleasing parents, teachers, supervisors. Residency directors. Medical directors. Admissions counselors. Compliance officers. Nursing managers. Supervisors. In order to get to where I am today, I became the perpetual professional "yes-woman."

In the process of trying to please everyone, I became paralyzed and incapable even of being able to say no. While this was something I worked on in my personal life, I found myself struggling with the ability to succeed in giving myself the permission to enforce the same boundaries in my professional life.

Speaking with mentors, friends, and colleagues, I found this problem to be ubiquitous and insidious. Is it because I feel privileged to be where I am? Is it a construct of how I actually got here? These questions have left me struggling, grappling with the post-decision wheel of regret, dreading, justifying, and acquiescence.

It is so easy to get caught up in the academic rigor of doing more with less and quickly. Take on committee assignments for credibility, not compensation. Say yes while hoping that an honest no would have been the answer instead.

But as I challenge and empower myself to pursue professional happiness and fulfillment, I embrace the challenge to be honest. To say yes to what serves me, my career, and my interests. To say no when it doesn't. To think first, decide, and avoid the constant replay of "what if I had answered differently."

I wish I could end this essay with a story of success and evoke the feeling of achievement and confidence that women in medicine—and in all fields—have earned and deserved. I don't think I have that yet.

I do, though, know where to look for inspiration. I have a community of women and mentors and friends who have fought that fight valiantly. They have emerged victorious, ready to tackle the next challenge on the road to professional fulfillment and success. I am grateful and will continue to work hard to follow in their footsteps as I forge my own path.

I Can't Do It All

Avital O'Glasser, MD, FACP, SFHM, DFPM

I don't know how you do it all.

It was a recent conversation—several recent conversations, actually.

I don't know how you do it all.

You must not sleep at night.

I used to demurely smile, emit a petite giggle, and say, "Thank you for that compliment." I used to continue to secure the reputation that I was able to do it all, indeed, to secure the illusion that I ran on caffeine, could run a 5-minute mile, and had a supra-physiologic ability to subsist on less than 2 hours of sleep a night.

"Well, since you mentioned it, I just somehow got it all done."

At some point in my journey, I realized that I was only hurting myself if I continued to pursue attainment of that external validation. And when I realized that it was humanly impossible to pursue and achieve the do-it-all endpoint, I then realized it was disingenuous to maintain the vanity of that mirage. Was the comment *I don't know how you do it all* a backhanded compliment? Was it wishful thinking? Was it a challenge? Was the pressure to maintain an impossible standard worsening the feelings of inadequacy and imposter syndrome in myself and others? It was exhausting—and inauthentic—to continue to put on a happy face and keep up appearances that I was indeed doing it all.

For too long, the culture of medicine has insisted that we are superhuman and that self-care is a sign of weakness. Doing it all is an impossible standard. It's an unhealthy standard. It's a dangerous standard. Pre-pandemic—and even after two years of this pandemic—we propagate a culture of working sick days, of not taking our vacation time, of catching up on work on weekends. We propagate a culture that we must devote as much of the 365 days in a year to work-related energy expenditure.

And then let's talk about the expectation that we possess the time-bending ability to cram far more than twenty-four hours of energy expenditure into only twenty-four hours. We add on the mounting daily workloads during our "first shift"[24] and the "second shift"[25] of family and home responsibilities including childcare. And we are then further expected to contour the time-space continuum to cram in the "third shift" of diversity and equity work,[26] and the "fourth shift" of ongoing advocacy and volunteerism in response to the COVID-19 pandemic.[27] Then add on all the additional bandwidth requirements we faced in 2022. By my calculations, that leaves . . . four hours to sleep at night. And even if you truly can run on four hours of sleep a night—WHY are we doing this to ourselves?

24 Silver, Julie. "The Pandemic Has Created a 4th Shift for Women in Medicine." Bench Press, 29 Mar. 2021, https://mgriblog.org/2021/03/30/the-pandemic-has-created-a-4th-shift-for-women-in-medicine

25 Hochchild, Arlie and Anne Machung. Second Shift: Working Families and the Revolution at Home. Penguin Books, 2012.

26 Santhosh Lekshmi, et al. "The "Third Shift": A Path Forward to Recognizing and Funding Gender Equity Efforts." Journal of Womens Health (Larchmt). vol. 29, no. 11, 29 Nov 2020, pp 1359-60. doi: 10.1089/jwh.2020.8679.

27 Silver, Julie. "The Pandemic Has Created a 4th Shift for Women in Medicine." Bench Press, 29 Mar. 2021, https://mgriblog.org/2021/03/30/the-pandemic-has-created-a-4th-shift-for-women-in-medicine

I can't do it all. I can't see patients, and lead a clinic, and serve on multiple COVID-response related committees . . . and also care for my family, and engage in self-care, and have time for my passions and fill-the-cup activities. If I find myself resorting to being sleep-deprived, skipping healthy meals, ordering take-out multiple times a week, not exercising, maxing out shortcuts, and burning the candle on both ends—if I find myself saying no to myself too often—then I need to start saying no to other things.

I have learned to advocate for extended deadlines, to ask for help, to delegate, to triage, and to sponsor. I have learned to set out-of-offices and avoid answering emails on nights and weekends. I have learned to just say no. I am learning to role model this and respond,

"I really DON'T do it all. I set boundaries, I prioritize, and I strive to say yes or no intentionally and authentically based on needs, responsibilities, impact, passions, and available creative energy."

I don't want to do it all.

I don't want to be known for doing it all.

I can't do it all.

I shan't do it all.

I won't do it all.

All the Christmas Activities

COL Cristin Mount, MD

It was a beautiful, sunny, Saturday morning. Spread out in front of me was a December calendar and twenty-five, tiny, hand-made cards representing different Holiday Activities, things like "Hot Cocoa," "Grinch Party," and "Watch 'Snowy Day.'" A mug of coffee sat to my left, the kids had music on in the background, and between intermittent dinosaur roars and "Mommy! He took my car!" I stared at two other calendars. One calendar was our work calendar, the other our generic home/school calendar. It was time to plan The Holiday Activities, a process I started two years ago to better ensure we were able to cram everything in and create Meaningful Memories and Traditions.

Christmas has long been my favorite holiday season. Traditions grounded in holidays were important when I was growing up as the oldest child of a military family. Much of our lives changed on an every-two-or-three-year basis, so joyous traditions held special importance. Putting the tree up on Christmas Eve happened whether we were in Texas or Germany. It represented consistency and roots in a way that "normal things" like hometowns, lifelong best friends, and the same school could not.

Three years ago, we entered that period where kids remember Christmas fun with expectations and anticipation. Ignoring the fact that both of us are full-time physicians and Army officers with significant work obligations that don't abate in December, I was determined to Make Meaningful Memories for our three small boys. It was a hectic mess. Supremely capable of multitasking at work and multitasking the usual home management burden, I felt that the added pressure of Making Meaningful Memories was just too much. Activities that should have been fun became chores, rushed into the space between the end of the workday and bedtime. Even worse, I had created Martha-Stewart-level expectations for myself.

Why, of course I can MAKE and decorate beautiful sugar cookies in between breastfeeding a two-month-old and taking an ICU call. And yes, I can absolutely make DIY Christmas "things" to hand out to work friends and colleagues. No problem!

My husband wisely helped where I'd let him. I ended that Christmas season exhausted, having not really enjoyed myself at all.

My entire professional life as an Intensivist boils down to bringing order to chaos. When things are a mess, I fix them. By system. So, the next year, I laid out All The Activities, labeled on tiny, handmade cards, and mapped them onto a calendar. Now I knew when we were going to Zoo Lights, when cookies should be baked, and when I could shop. Bonus, at least now my husband could anticipate when I was going to push myself too far in the effort to Make Meaningful Memories. I was finally able to take it down a notch or two and not crawl out of bed on the 26th wondering what I had just put myself through.

Here I am now, buoyed by my success, on a Saturday in mid-November, balancing coffee, "Get off your brother!" and now

THREE calendars. The first thing I did on the Activities Map was pencil in my work schedule. *OOF? 26 November through 18 December in the ICU and only two days off. Who the heck did that?* (Cue me, reminding myself that I must learn to say no.) Then I penciled in my husband's schedule and the school schedule. Now to balance The Activities across this map. We usually like to put up our Christmas tree the first weekend in December, but I'm working nights that weekend, so that won't work. We want to go to our local Zoo Lights but need a weeknight (so it isn't too busy) where both of us are home, not on-call, and can get there when it opens. This was going to be hard! I realized that many things I obligate myself to do each year aren't even on the Activities list. How was I going to get those done too? I took a deep breath and muttered to myself,

What if we DON'T do All The Activities?

Shocked that the mere thought didn't induce panic, I moved to the second-best thing I do as an Intensivist—cutting out the unnecessary stuff. Like discontinuing polypharmacy in a geriatric septic patient, I eyed those tiny cards and started discarding Activities that weren't going to make the cut this year. I gave myself permission—actually, I finally listened to my husband who had been encouraging me for years to give myself permission—to scale down. Do what I felt was essential for Making Meaningful Memories, things I truly enjoyed, or the kids truly enjoyed, and let the rest go. I identified the things that were super easy for one parent to do: "Dance Party," "Snowman Pancakes," or things I could count twice like the school Christmas Program night that is now tagged as "Singing Christmas Songs." No DIY gifts for colleagues and friends. Gift cards for out-of-town family members are just fine this year. I'm not going to cook from scratch a large meal for my husband's fellowship Christmas party; thus, the Christmas CrockPotLuck has been born. We're still going to make bird feeders and drink hot chocolate. The tree and the decorations will go up at some point. I may just buy the Christmas cookies this year.

My goal over the next few weeks is to give myself some grace. Cut myself some slack. I'm going to focus on the reason for creating tradition, to help our kids feel that they have something special, something they can say is "ours." Making Meaningful Memories matters, but only if the process is free of unreasonable expectations.

So, I'm sitting here now with an altered list, a lighter calendar, fewer tasks, and more time. Giving myself permission to NOT do All The Activities may be the best gift I receive this year.

Navigating Complexities of Work-Life Balance*

Maryam Beheshti Lustberg, MD, MPH

It was a cold, Thursday night in November—the night of Thanksgiving 2022.

The driver opened the trunk, put my suitcase in, and I got into the car. We were on our way to John F. Kennedy Airport, about 2 hours away. I was going to take the longest flight of my life—fifteen hours to South Korea. I was leaving on a Thursday night after having said goodbye to my family at our Thanksgiving dinner and I planned to arrive Saturday morning in Seoul. Work-life balance felt very off-kilter to me as I rode away.

Mom Guilt

In the days leading up to this trip, when people asked me about my Thanksgiving plans, I would consistently get the surprised look when they said, "You are going to Korea?" followed by, "You are so amazing, I don't know how you do it." or "Are you excited?"

The truth was that as I was on my way to the airport, I felt anything but amazing or excited. I kept asking myself what I was doing and is this really how I should be spending my holiday weekend.

I am the mom of a nine-year-old boy, a breast medical oncologist, chief of breast medical oncology at Yale Cancer Center, and president of the international society of Multinational Association of Cancer in Supportive Care (MASCC).

The Korean Cancer Supportive Society had recently joined as an affiliate to MASCC, and as president, I had the opportunity to travel to South Korea to give a plenary talk and officially celebrate the collaboration between the societies. The festivities fell during our holiday weekend. American Thanksgiving is clearly not a global holiday.

By the time I arrived at the airport, I had allowed mom guilt to saturate me thoroughly. It was time to deal with the practicalities of international travel by getting through the airport to my gate. It was the first time I was flying business class and I began to relax in the comfort of the Korean Air lounge. I was tired and anxious but was also beginning to feel the inklings of excitement over the wonderful privilege and opportunity that this was.

Compromise

I arrived on a Saturday morning and began to experience a beautiful new land unknown to me previously.

I spoke to my son, who told me proudly I was talking to him from the future given the time zone difference. I was in the future and the tethering of my old negative thought patterns including feelings of guilt and anxieties seemed a part of the past.

I met with colleagues, signed the affiliation agreement as president, and gave my talk. The evening ended with a soothing traditional Korean meal in a restaurant that was previously inhabited by a member of the royal family. My hosts were sure to point out that I was sitting in a chair previously sat on by Pope Francis. The surreal evening ended with an exchange of thoughtful gifts, including a stamp with my name in Korean. I left dinner knowing that I will fondly remember this night for years to come.

The next day was my only free day in Seoul before my flight back home on Monday. The work-life debate once again took hold. This version was about whether to spend the day working and catching up on all the backlog of items on my to do list. I knew if I worked all day that I would feel less stressed the rest of week. Yet, the idea of not seeing some of the key historic sites in South Korea after such a long plane ride seemed like such a loss. So, I compromised with myself and booked a half-day tour. My plan was to work the rest of the day.

On the tour, I visited traditional Korean temples and palaces. I felt more alive and nimbler than I had felt in a very long time. With me were a small group of Americans, who were also there for work as a tightly knit group of colleagues. As I heard their easy banter, one conversation line stood out to me for its simplicity and absence of guilt. They asked each other what day they celebrated Thanksgiving so that they could spend time with friends and family since they were unable to be home on the actual holiday. It may seem obvious to some to do this. I had certainly heard of these types of modifications before, but in that moment I realized that I had torn myself apart with guilt and anxiety over being away when there was an alternative mode of thinking and being. I felt happy about the opportunity of this enriching experience and for my current leadership roles that allowed me the chance to experience it.

Navigating Life's Complexities

I ended up extending the tour to a full day. The day continued to calm my heart as I walked down winding streets, tasted food in open air markets, and found items to take back to my family, including a snow globe for my son. He has accumulated a collection of these of all the places I have visited for my work. He is proud of me and my many accomplishments.

Ultimately, I don't have answers for the complexities we navigate as professionals with personal lives that all need tending. After this trip, I realized that one-size prescriptive recommendations of "just say no" or "family first" don't always resonate. It is possible to travel to a foreign land on the night of Thanksgiving and return more enriched and clearer about the beauty of life and connections.

I hugged my nine-year-old son on Monday night and all was full circle again.

* This piece comes from the partnership between the WIMS Blog and the Healio Women in Oncology blog:Lustberg M. Women in Oncology (blog): Navigating complexities of work-life balance. Healio, December 23, 2022. Available at: https://www.healio.com/news/hematology-oncology/20221223/blog-navigating-complexities-of-worklife-balance. Reprinted with permission from Healio.

The Gift of Bandwidth

Avital O'Glasser, MD, FACP, SFHM, DFPM

I'm generally not one for New Year's resolutions. New Year's reflections? *Yes.* New Year's hopes? *Yes.* New Year's intentions? *Yes.*

But as I crossed from 2022 into 2023, I did articulate a New Year's resolution.

I resolved to give myself, and others, the gift of bandwidth—the capacity (physically, mentally, or emotionally) to handle tasks and challenges.

Over the last decade, my identity—and the many hats I wear at any given moment—has depended on the externally imposed expectation that I must *be busy*.

I must *be busy* as a clinician: *can't justify that unfilled patient appointment slot!*

I must *be busy* as a clinic leader: *no taking thirty seconds to trim a hangnail during the work day!*

I must *be busy* as an academic clinician: *better be working on that research data set instead of taking a coffee break!*

I must *be busy* as a mom and a partner. Anytime someone asked how work, home life, or I was doing personally, the answer was always an automatic, "It's busy." The pressure was externally *AND* internally imposed.

I've embraced the tenet that I can't do it all and that to maintain the facade that I *AM* doing it all was a disingenuous and damaging precedent to role-model. Other amazing voices have written similarly themed posts. But what was the next leap? How does one go from setting boundaries to reinforcing boundaries to actively creating more bandwidth?

I'm a planner—I keep to-do lists and block my work time during the week so that I can maximize focused attention on tasks, both administrative and creative. It's my attempt to stay on track during the week and minimize multitasking as much as possible. However, as 2022 came to a close, I realized that I was still over-scheduling myself too much—not in a two-meetings-at-once kind of way but that every minute of the day was scripted and scheduled. I think this was very much driven by academic expectations that salaried time (academic time, leadership time) to not see patients was a precious "gift" that needed to be fulfilled down to the very last second to appease the bestowers of said funded, protected time: *Like Pandora entrusted with the jar, don't you dare let an unfilled minute of time slip away from you!* Even "flow time" felt hard to justify. But when every moment of the day is scripted and budgeted, there is no flexibility for being responsive and dynamic. So, I was still multitasking day in and day out. I was answering Teams messages while on meetings; I was racing through projects to find ten minutes to thoughtfully answer an email; and I was groaning when an urgent meeting got added to my calendar displacing my anticipated time to update a lecture. I didn't like how I had set myself up for frustration by doing the work I love to do and find fulfilling, because it involves the power of relationships and connection. My virtual "open door policy" was leading to banging my head on my physical desk.

I realized that I needed to give myself permission to have the bandwidth to be available.

My leadership position as a clinic medical director and my personal leadership style involves being receptive and responsive. This is NOT an example of being beholden to "your lack of planning *IS* my emergency." Instead, the reality of my work is that I need to be available often on very short notice. I need to be available, accessible, *AND* present. Creating more bandwidth to be available does *NOT* mean I'm lowering boundaries; rather, I am repositioning them to improve the architecture of my days and weeks.

So yes, I resolved to give myself, and others, the gift of my bandwidth. That entailed that I fiercely, passionately, and proactively protect existing bandwidth. And it entailed seeking ways to gain more bandwidth, such as crossing off thirty minutes to update a talk on a Tuesday's to-do list in order to . . . in order to "*BE.*" Or to postpone a nonurgent project when time-sensitive tasks arise the Friday afternoon going into a long weekend.

I recognize that the external pressures imposed on many might make such a plan challenging or impossible, and I acknowledge that my very own ability to set this intention comes from some place of privilege. But, I hope others will *seek* more bandwidth as well—even in the times when it feels impossible.

Seek it.

Three Women in Oncology Look Forward to Running the 126th Boston Marathon*

Amy Comander, MD, DipABLM;
Gabriela Hobbs, MD; Sahdna Vora, MD

Inspire. Empower. Celebrate!

These words were the slogan for the 126th running of the Boston Marathon, which aimed to recognize and honor the 50th anniversary of the 1972 race that featured the first women's division in race history. In 1972, eight women met the qualifying standard and were made official entrants to the marathon. Five of those original women celebrated in Boston on race day, which was April 18, 2022, and we were thrilled that the three of us—Comander, Hobbs, and Vora—ran in that anniversary race.

The three of us, busy juggling our demanding, important jobs, our parenting responsibilities and care for our families—all during the pandemic—ran in the footsteps of those original eight trailblazers. Each of us has found that during the pandemic, running was not only an important way to get exercise but also an opportunity to focus on our own self-care, build resilience, and develop meaningful connections with each other.

Des Linden, winner of the 2018 Boston Marathon women's race, stated: "Remember your *why*. When things get hard you have the decision to bail, or you can remember your 'why.'"[28] Below, each of us share "why" we ran the 2022 Boston Marathon.

Sadhna R. Vora, MD: Inspire!

Running helps me put challenges into perspective, gives me a sense of mental clarity, and helps me find joy in nature, even on those dark, New England-winter mornings! It makes me feel stronger, both physically and mentally, and I bring that into my day-to-day life.

Not only does running help me feel more grounded, it also provides a community, connecting me with other runners like my fellow authors Amy and Gaby.

Lastly, running for a good cause provides that extra burst of energy when I need it the most, and I felt fortunate to be able to contribute by doing something I love! This was my first marathon, and I ran it in support of Massachusetts General Hospital Pediatric Oncology.

Gabriela Hobbs, MD: Empower!

Most of my day is filled with parenting and work responsibilities as an oncologist. I love being a mom and an oncologist. Both demand a lot from me in a good way!

Each morning while everyone in my house is asleep, I lace up—and layer up—and head out for a run. Each run helps to balance my thoughts, clears my work-related concerns, and gets me ready for the day. No matter how hectic a day may be, I always feel better

---

28 Boston Marathon Pro. ""Remember your why. When things get hard you have the decision to bail or you can remember your why." -@des_linden #MondayMotivation". Twitter. July 8, 2020. https://twitter.com/Boston26_2_Pro/status/1016326693882073088?s=20

knowing I've accomplished something before the day has started. I'm always able to give more to others knowing I've dedicated that peaceful sunrise hour to myself.

Running also gives me community, which was especially critical during the isolating pandemic years. It was through running that I was able to make some amazing friends and run my first marathon. Amy was my personal course director for my first marathon during the pandemic. Through Amy, I was able to connect with Sadhna who was getting ready to run her first marathon!

That year, I was thrilled to run on behalf of my father who has retinitis pigmentosa and to raise money for Massachusetts Eye and Ear Hospital in support of their research efforts for this disease.

Amy Comander, MD, DipABLM: Celebrate!

For the past nine years, I have been fortunate to run the Boston Marathon for charitable causes. This year, I was honored to run in support of the Ellie Fund, a nonprofit organization that provides essential support for those receiving treatment for breast cancer in Massachusetts.

In February 2021, a piece I wrote was published in *The Oncologist* about my reflections on running the Boston Marathon during the pandemic.[29] While preparing for the 2022 race, I reflected further on these running lessons: *purpose, resilience,* and *gratitude.*

When it comes to *purpose,* I think of my patients and the challenges they face during treatment for cancer. It is my honor to run in support of my patients. I dedicate each mile to them and to my mother who died from an aggressive cancer in 2011.

---

29 Comander, Amy. "Remember Your Why: An Oncologist's Reflections on Running During the COVID-19 Pandemic." *Oncologist.* vol. 26, no. 4, 2021 Apr, pp. 348-9. doi: 10.1002/onco.13683.

When it comes to *resilience,* we all had a crash course navigating uncertainty during the pandemic. Who taught me the most about this important skill? My patients. Individuals undergoing cancer treatment faced unprecedented challenges over the first two years of the pandemic.

Finally, when it comes to *gratitude,* I am fortunate to have a meaningful and rewarding job as a breast oncologist and to learn from my patients who have taught me the true meaning of Amby Burfoot's running mantra: "Every mile out there is a gift, and every finish line is a gift." These lessons helped me navigate and celebrate those 26.2 miles! I was also incredibly grateful to run alongside Sadhna and Gaby.

The three of us looked forward to that historic race day. We were inspired by those original eight women; we hoped to empower others to discover the joy from running; and most importantly, we celebrated as we cross that finish line in Copley Square!

"Running rewards consistency and resilience.
So does life. Keep showing up."
—DES LINDEN

* This piece comes from the partnership between the WIMS Blog and the Healio Women in Oncology blog:*
Comander A, Hobbs G and Vora SR. Women in Oncology (blog): Three women in oncology look forward to running the 126th Boston Marathon. Healio, April 12, 2022. Available at: https://www.wimedicine.org/blog/ three-women-in-oncology-look-forward-to-running-the-126th-boston- marathon. Reprinted with permission from Healio.

From the Tennis Court to the Operating Room: How My Experience as a Camp Counselor Prepared Me to Be an Orthopaedic Surgeon

Jennifer M. Weiss, MD

In 2021, women continued to make up less than ten percent of practicing orthopaedic surgeons in the US.[30] I made the decision to pursue a career in this male-dominated profession at the age of twenty-four. I was young and fearless. I am getting older and I am trying to reach back to my twenty-four-year-old self to understand who I was and what made me think that it was a good idea to immerse myself in the challenge of surrounding myself with mostly men. This summer I have had time to reflect as I have returned to the place where I spent my summers during those influential years.

During college, I spent two summers as a counselor at a sports camp in the Berkshire Mountains of Massachusetts. The camp initially opened in the 1910s as a boys camp. In the late 1980s, the

30 Orthopaedic Practice in the U.S. 2018. AAOS Department of Clinical Quality and Value. January 2019.

camp opened to girls. In 1991, there was a small girls camp, making up about ten percent of the campers and counselors, embedded within the boys camp. That was my first summer as a tennis counselor. Of the fifteen tennis counselors, I was the only woman.

I had to prove myself as an athlete every day. But every evening I went back to my cabin full of young women and these female counselors and campers were pure fun. Many were fierce athletes. Some were not. Some were artistic or brainy, and the crew was a motley one. The thing we all had in common was fast friendship and loyalty—we knew how to stick together.

I made some unlikely friends that summer. My co-counselor was a fast talking, incredibly intelligent woman. She had big, Long Island-hair. I learned immediately that NO ONE messed with her. She gave me a once over when I arrived, unimpressed with my Williams College Lacrosse T-shirt, ripped up jeans, and Birkenstocks. Her hair was perfectly curled and her scrunchy socks matched her tank top. She was fun and established. It was clear that she was in charge, both socially and in her job description.

One of my best friends from high school joined me. She had just finished her sophomore year at Duke. She was a great soccer player and was unfazed by being the only woman among the male soccer staff. We also met a soft-spoken Midwesterner who worked on the waterfront. She and I came from different parts of the country, from different kinds of families, but we had so much in common. We were bits of calm in the storm. We were quick to help, we worked hard, and we both fell in love with summer boyfriends. We did not think to push on the male hierarchy entrenched in decades of history and tradition. We did not know then who we would become.

I returned to the camp in 2016. My oldest daughter was a camper. One of my campers had married one of the counselors from my 1990s version of camp, and their daughter and mine became fast friends. The director of the waterfront was the same old guy, with the only real change in 25 years being the loss of his blond, wild, mane of hair. So many of my people were still there. And I joined for a week as the camp doctor. In 2017, the camp celebrated its 100th birthday. Campers and counselors from far and wide returned, including my former co-counselers.

One had put her articulate strength to use. She is now the mayor of her town in Florida. The other is a tenured professor at a university in Indiana. And the three of us agreed that our experience at this camp was a huge influence on our professional success.

It turns out that spending a summer in close quarters in a male-dominated environment might have been the best preparation for orthopaedics. There was no fear in competing with the men around me. I learned to separate myself from the behavior that was not interesting to me. I established boundaries. More importantly, I learned to believe that I could do things differently but just as well as the men surrounding me as I learned not to be intimidated. Probably the most important thing that these summers taught me was the meaning of a small tribe of women in a huge sea of boys and men steeped in tradition.

In 2021, the camp is almost half girls and women. The women counselors include top athletes from basketball to softball to soccer. The stands for girls' sports are filled by boys cheering, just like the girls cheer for the boys. The color-war teams are led by a male and a female general each season. The girls and women are no longer a small minority among a male-led majority. In 2021, I spent two weeks watching my two daughters inhabit a world that is teaching them gender equality in athletics and in life.

Chapter 3

BURNT-OUT IMPOSTERS

Burnout

Ami K. Naik, MD

Physician burnout has been brought to the forefront thanks to the COVID-19 pandemic. It has given us, as female physicians, a platform to address our thoughts, opinions, and experiences of gaining our rightful place in the world of medicine. Physician burnout in females used to hide in the shadows of misogyny and "tradition," but we are now open, honest, and fighting back on the idea that being a physician means sacrificing other things that bring joy and meaning to our lives.

I have come to the conclusion, however, that it is not just physician burnout that is the crux of the issue. It is what I term "human burnout." What is human burnout? It is the collective feeling of not just being burned out in our professional lives, but also feeling burned out from our spouses, our partners, our children, our friends, our society, and even our pets. How do we get to this point? We keep giving and giving while those around us keep taking and taking. Then, one day, there is a straw that breaks the camel's back, as they say. It's one small thing—a request from a friend to go to another fundraiser, another activity our child wants to be in, or coming home to our pets jumping on us because no one has fed them yet—when we suddenly, like flipping a switch, stop caring.

Our minds go numb because we cannot handle one more thing. Our thought processes shut down. We are tired. This fatigue is not relieved with a good night's sleep. This fatigue begins deep in our cores and expands outward to where we barely have the energy to put one foot in front of the other. It sweeps over us like a heavy fog, dulling our senses, and creating doubt about whether we took the fork in the road of life that was right for us. It shuts down our synapses so that all we want to do, and all we can do, is just be. That's it—just be. We don't want to walk, talk, or think. It is hard enough keeping our blood flowing, our lungs breathing, and our hearts beating. It feels as though we are jellyfish, where that internal structure that grounds us has collapsed. The collective taking from our life reservoirs leave us empty. There is taking but there is no replenishing. We are somehow supposed to keep giving without the time, energy, or ability to refuel. No one thinks about our need to be refilled. And so we are left empty. When we are empty, we shut down.

We are all supposed to be the proverbial Wonder Woman. We are expected to do everything, give everything, solve problems, take care of everyone else's happiness as well as be kind, courteous, gracious, and respectful all of the time. Yet, when we try with all our hearts and souls to do these things, our intentions, our ideas, our thought processes are still questioned. We are not allowed to be sick, have a bad day, sleep in on a Saturday morning, express our frustrations without judgment or be angry. And the most important thing is that we cannot say no. If the word no escapes from our lips, the first question that is asked is *"What is wrong with you?"*

This question is the ultimate question, the sum of all that we are supposedly doing wrong being defined as an inherent flaw in

us. We are the problem. We are the issue. The paradox is just that—
that we are the problem and the solution. This emptiness that we
feel at our cores cannot be attributed to anxiety or depression. This
goes much deeper. Our life energy resides in our cores, the place
where we store our identity and our purpose. And when these
cores are depleted, we lose ourselves to the whims of everyone else
until we are a meaningless empty shell.

So, make sure you refill and nourish your core. Without it
being strong and full, we cannot be the best versions of ourselves.
What is your core? It's the place where you keep your inner peace.
It's the place where you hold your most precious and sacred memories. It's the place where your soul comes to find rest and replen-
ishment. It's the place where your hopes and dreams for the future
take shape. How do you nourish and refill it? It's not something
that you can solely rely on other people to do. That's not to say
that others in your life won't contribute to this nourishment. They
will cook dinner for you, let you sleep in on your day off, gift you a
massage gift card, or just sit and listen to the ups and downs of your
day. This will partially replenish you. But this is not enough. The
way that you nourish and fill yourself is to live your life guided by
your values. To do this, you must do something that has the potential to be very hard and painful but ultimately can result in the opportunity to mold and shape your life the way you want it to be. You
must recognize your values. Sharing your precious and finite time,
expressing your love, learning something new, giving your body
(your temple) a rest, and bringing joy to someone else's life are a
few examples of "giving" values that we can hold. Examples of "receiving" values are acquiring wealth, working up the healthcare hierarchy, buying material things, and traveling to exotic places. None

of these values are right or wrong. In fact, most of our values are a complex mixture of all of the above plus some. The question you must ask yourself is, "What brings joy and freedom to my heart?" Is it spending time with your family, learning a new craft, expressing your love for animals by volunteering at your local shelter, being able to fund your child's 529 college account, traveling to Tahiti, or a mixture of all of the above? Once you identify your values, you can then portion the circle that is your life with those values and how much importance you give to each of them. That circle will end up looking like a pie cut into uneven triangles as you decide what you give more or less weight to. You then live your life guided by these values. This nourishes and refills your core. Without a strong core, we cannot be the best versions of ourselves.

No More Lip Service: Let's All Advocate for Physician Wellness

Trintje Johansson, DO

Medical school and residency selection have changed to value humanism and compassion more than in years past, changing how we practice medicine and who makes up the people practicing medicine. Many early career physicians and trainees wish to pursue mental health care as a part of remaining healthy so they can provide compassionate and humanistic care. But then they find themselves thrust into a situation where doing so can impact their credentialing and licensure.

There are lots of reasons why physicians don't seek mental health care, including but not limited to the fear of having to report receiving mental health care. There is also stigma that to have a mental health diagnosis or to seek counseling is a weakness. Women are also more likely to be penalized or seen as weak for seeking help. We can help to normalize help-seeking by actively and publicly sharing resources that provide mental health care to clinicians, such as Emotional PPE (personal protective equipment), the Physician Support Line, the Helping Healthcare Heal Coalition at the Institute for Healthcare Improvement (IHI), professional society resources, or their employee assistance program, and having content on physician mental health during meetings such as grand rounds. But none of these fully address someone's fears, including women's, about having to report mental health on their license or credentialing applications.

Physicians who are concerned about having to report receiving mental health care are not fully wrong about it. Historically, most state licensing boards and healthcare institutions have stigmatized physicians who have sought mental health care. The good news is that this is changing, and many states are changing their application processes so that they are only asking about receiving mental health care or having a mental health diagnosis if it affects how they provide care. Some notable examples of states with recent changes are South Dakota, Arizona, New Mexico, and Minnesota. Even more states are evaluating their processes in response to recommendations from national organizations not to ask these questions. Many other states are doing so because there is now a more widespread recognition that practicing medicine in a pandemic is hard, and the adage that no one can give from an empty cup has never been truer.

Progress in revising organization credentialing applications is generally lagging. Most healthcare institutions have been overwhelmed for the last several years and have not yet reexamined their internal processes despite people in those same organizations advocating for state license application changes. But this, too, can change, and *you* can be a part of this change.

Often, hospitals and health systems have not had anyone ask them to change! If you have a moment, you can reach out to your credentialing office (sometimes called a medical staff office) and ask them to evaluate their applications.

During a hard time, it can be hard to consider doing *one more thing*. This is true! It is also true that sometimes a small amount of effort can do a lot of good. In this case one example of that is asking your organization to revise their credential application to not ask about mental health care and to add language that is supportive of clinicians receiving mental health care.

The Healer's Search

Namrata Ragade, MD, CPCC, ACC

Here and there
We rush each day
Looking for that elusive
Somewhere, something
At times we need
To sit and stare
Reflect what matters
To our heart
And listen to what it says . . .

Then we can find joy
And we can cry
Let go of what matters not
Bring in what we care about
Laugh and dance a little each day
We are human and need that self-care

We are love, we know that
Exhausted and overwhelmed
We forget that . . .

We yearn to find the happy spark
The one that lights our thoughts
Hidden, yet always there
Seek and it will reveal itself!

Resiliency, Burnout, and Wellness in Medicine

Aishwarya Thapliyal, MD

The best way to find yourself is to lose yourself
in the service of others.

—MAHATMA GANDHI

The healthcare industry around the globe is committed to providing quality medical facilities to its citizens, and the executors of these facilities make this possible. The context of the conversation is the healthcare providers who dedicate their lives for the sole purpose of helping others. The day you decide that medicine is your career of choice, the journey of perseverance begins. One can never show how much hard work is required every single day to sustain his or her position. The number of years and financial burden that an individual must bear to train and ultimately serve the public is outrageous. Fair wages are an issue in many countries, including the United States, and primarily affect resident physicians. The one who survives the storm is made to conquer it, which seems like an accurate description.

The American Medical Association (AMA) conducted an online survey published in 2020, indicating that 42% of physicians experience burnout.[31] Not surprisingly, female doctors are most affected. The results led me to think about whether or not the societal obligations or stereotypical "duties" of a woman, including motherhood and household management, have anything to do with her mental health decline. The gender and the racial pay gaps are other hurdles to solving this issue when the expectation of working hours and patient outcomes is the same.

The best advice that I received in med school was always to take care of your health to provide the best care to your patients; it's like the flight announcements: "wear your mask before helping others." In an article published by the *Canadian Medical Association Journal* in 2018, Alison Motluck says that, "physicians whose surveys revealed signs of burnout were 2.2 times as likely to report a perceived medical error."[32]

The great news is that the importance of mental health is getting the attention of people at-large, and healthcare providers are leading the way. The stigma is slowly dissolving, and more physicians are getting the help and medications that they genuinely need and deserve to take care of their health. Doctors should advocate for the same for everyone. Younger and newer generations are more open to getting mental health help and advocating for others.

In the end, what matters is the appreciation of the availability of the healthcare system in place. Taking advantage of these ser-

31 Berg, Sara. "Half of health workers report burnout amid COVID-19." AMA. July 20, 2021. https://www.ama-assn.org/practice-management/physician-health/half-health-workers-report-burnout-amid-covid-19

32 Motluk, Alison. "Do doctors experiencing burnout make more errors?" *Canadian Medical Association Journal.* vol. 190, no. 40, Oct 2018, pp E1216-1217. https://www.ncbi.nlm.nih.gov/pmc/articles/PMC6175626/

vices should not only be seen as a need but a right, especially for women experiencing burnout. The world needs more examples and success stories, which are only possible with participation and openness, especially by healthcare physicians, and by including empowered woman voices. The medical field is a tiny and well-connected community with support pouring in from different parts of the world. This contribution can only strengthen our stance on mental health advocacy and help eliminate the stigma surrounding it. You and I are a part of this system; our responsibility is to build trust and strive for wellness, an epitome of a bright future.

Chapter 4
COMMUNITY

The Power of @PelotonMed

Deanna Behrens, MD

Like many others during the initial stages of the pandemic, I craved something to replace the community that I normally found in person, at work and church, and with friends and family. I also realized that I wanted to use the time to do something positive and meaningful for myself during what was an exceedingly difficult and uncertain time.

Luckily, I had previously turned to social media, specifically Twitter, in late 2016 and early 2017 after the 2016 presidential election. This period of transition was in some ways similar to the time in the spring and summer of 2020. I needed an outlet to connect with other health care providers and to achieve a sense of purpose by advocating for my vulnerable patient population. I formed genuine relationships with people in #WomenInMedicine, #tweetiatrician, and #PedsICU. They provided invaluable support and mentorship.

At the start of 2020, I knew that I needed an outlet for all my energy and anxiety during that upcoming spring, and I wanted to use it to become healthier and stronger. Peloton was something vague to me. Friends and colleagues at work had talked about the value they received from a community formed around exercise; it was more than a bike to them.

Getting a Peloton is a big commitment financially. Would I use it? Would I like it? How would it help me get through the pandemic? I started to notice #PelotonMedTwitter around that time and followed a few friends who had one. I decided to start with the app, which is something I recommend to anyone who is contemplating the bike. I loved the instructors, and I loved the energy. I was ready for the bike. Out of an overabundance of optimism, I decided to join Dr. Gretchen Winter on a ride. It was my first and her 200th.

One of the hallmarks of the company is the social aspect—which especially blossomed during the isolation of the pandemic when we could not go to our usual gyms. You can have friends and give high fives. You celebrate milestone rides and exercise streaks. You can train using the same program as those around you and get badges for completing them. There is a leaderboard. The instructors say that the most important thing about the leaderboard is showing up, and some people do compete only against themselves. But for some, there is a friendly rivalry that pushes everyone to do better.

I did not create the hashtag #PelotonMedTwitter—all the credit goes to Nicole Salvatore for that. But I did start a peloton med challenge, and thus @PelotonMed was created. Someone asked me later if I was surprised how the account grew. During that specific time (early pandemic) and with that specific demographic (anyone even tangentially related to healthcare who was interested in Peloton), it felt like an organic continuation of the community that had already been established. It made sense that there is a significant overlap in the Venn diagram between people who turn to social exercise groups and health care providers who turn to social media to connect, learn, and educate.

Shortly after starting the account, I asked Gretchen if she would be interested in co-leading it with me. Though it is a light-hearted account, we do take it seriously. It means something to the people who are part of it. We want to offer a place that is supportive and inclusive. We are deeply aware that the cost can be prohibitive, and so we always emphasize that you do not need the equipment to participate; while we call ourselves @PelotonMed, any form of exercise counts. A big rule—our only rule, really—is that we do not tolerate people who disrespect or put down others. Everyone is welcome, and we have doctors, nurses, dieticians, therapists, child life specialists, statisticians, medical librarians, and even a financial specialist who works with physicians. From the beginning, it was about community not competitiveness.

Every person who participates in @PelotonMed enriches it. Sometimes we interact with the company's official social media account (@onepeloton), sometimes with instructors, and memo-rably, John Foley himself once helped us. However, we are mostly a self-sufficient group. We have our own traditions and our own shorthand methods of communication. Dr. Ken Tegtmeyer is famous for his #FBHi5 (fly by high fives). We celebrate each other's pro-fessional accomplishments. We rooted for Gabby Brauner Librizzi during her journey through medical school and running her first marathon. We amplify and join in with @PelotonPHM, the pediatric hospital medicine group. We lift each other up and we hold each other accountable. We were even on an episode of Dr. Mark Shap-iro's podcast, *Explore the Space*, to speak about the unexpected but wonderful and supportive community we had built and nurtured.

Though I have not met the vast majority of those on @PelotonMed, I have made real friends through this experience. It has been an unexpected pleasure to meet #PelotonMedTwitter members at various conferences—although I was secretly jealous of those who got to meet in person at last year's "Women in Medicine Summit." Dr. Jessie Allan came by and gave me a real-life #FBHi5 at the Pediatric Academic Societies Meeting. It was a great delight to finally meet Gretchen in person when we were asked to be on a panel together at the Society of Critical Care Medicine conference. It was fitting that I met Gretchen on a panel about wellness and well-being, because being a member of a community, of this community, has been healing for me. It has helped me deal with complex emotions and to prioritize my own mental and physical health during the most challenging time in my career. I hope—and anticipate—that I am not alone in these reflections.

To Fit In or Not to Fit In

Sarah Bhagudas

While we hear stories of the Women in Medicine Summit being life-changing, it's nice to step back and look at the bigger picture or the WHY. I like to think of gender equity (or the lack thereof) as a giant picture puzzle with just the border pieces snapped in. This border is compiled of historical big-shot women. I'm talking about women at Ella Josephine Baker and Susan B. Anthony's level. They were the foundations amongst others. Next, you have women like Dr. Shikha Jain or Dr. Neelum Aggarwal, amongst *many* others, who are placing puzzle pieces down. The Summit gives us a place to be those puzzle pieces as well, filling in the rest of the picture.

I've been a part of the WIMS team since September 2021. I joined the virtual conference at a time when I felt like I needed to be fighting for a cause instead of doing nothing. It was a time when I was moving to a new country for medical school and things were all over the place mentally. Fast forward to this year, I joined the research team and threw myself into unfamiliar territory. I am a natural introvert and meeting new people, let alone incredibly powerful women, was something I typically would run from.

However, I became a student admin helping with anything I could do, just to say that I can help the Summit move forward in any way possible. I wanted to fit in a small role because I knew that was all I could do at this time as a medical student. Being on Zoom calls with women who were in ALL different types of fields and at the top of their careers was exhilarating but extremely intimidating to me, as a Caribbean medical student in Grenada. Imposter syndrome and I are one. It took time but I became very comfortable around the amazing philanthropy team over the months. When the opportunity to rotate in Chicago came around, I figured this was THE sign that everything was falling in place.

After signing up as a volunteer, I was nervous, excited, and scared, all at the same time. What if these women saw me in person and didn't take me seriously? Typing this, I laugh at the fact that I thought this at the time, because the Summit was made to break down questions like that. While packing my life up for Chicago a few days before the Summit, a great portion of my world turned upside down. I dealt with the loss of someone dear and it shook me. Amidst this, life does move on, and I had to move the day after this devastating loss. I was in Chicago—alone and mourning—about to go to a conference for the first time, a bit of a situation that I probably was not mentally ready for. Nevertheless, I was going to present my paper and represent my team as they deserved. It took everything in my power to peel myself off the bed the morning of Friday, September 16th. While I looked forward to seeing everybody, as I had for the entire year, I was not myself.

To say "fangirling" when I saw every person I followed on Twitter is an understatement. I was starstruck. These were my celebrities. I had the responsibility of helping with registration and

I am so glad I did. Let's just say it took all my professionalism not to ask for a picture with everybody I registered (*cough, cough* Dr. Jessi Gold). The hard thoughts became afterthoughts. It was almost emotional seeing everybody in person. No, not almost. I cried.

These were women whose thoughts on Twitter were retweeted and rejoiced in my personal life. Their articles were circulated at every chance I had. The intimidation I felt at the beginning slipped away throughout the day. Despite my recent loss, I didn't feel alone. By the time I did my poster presentation, there weren't roles or positions. I felt like these women were my comrades in this bigger fight that we all came here for. I felt an inner reward for simply being around them—like a gold star sticker on my soul. While I shall continue fangirling over everyone on Twitter until future WIMS, I take comfort for now knowing that I became a piece of a giant puzzle during the Summit, and I actually fit pretty nicely in it.

A New Take on Kitchen Cabinets–A Reflection of the 2021 Women in Medicine Summit

Mysa Abdelrahman

Where once the kitchen was synonymous with being the place of a woman, the 2021 Women in Medicine Summit challenged this narrative by engaging women in varying fields of medicine to empower their successors.

Dr. Ngozi Ezike started the incredible weekend by channeling the historical term "kitchen cabinet" for the modern context of having supportive people in our lives who help keep us grounded. Being a woman in medicine comes with its own unique set of challenges, whether it be balancing family and work responsibilities, combating harassment and bias, or promoting healthy work environments; it seems that the tasks women in medicine face are endless. Having a "kitchen cabinet" is therefore quintessential in being centered and moving forward in a meaningful way that promotes change and growth in our environments.

The 2021 Women in Medicine Summit has provided me with my own kitchen cabinet, who I look forward to learning from and growing with throughout my medical career.

Being a first-year medical student in the middle of a pandemic was no easy feat. Given that my curriculum had been fully online, the days seemed to be monotonous in nature, and I found exhaustion setting in much earlier than it would have pre-pandemic. Buried behind screens of varying sizes, interacting with classmates via Zoom, and not experiencing a hands-on medical education, I felt so far removed from the thing I was so adamant about studying not too long ago. The 2021 summit revitalized my intentions and reminded me that the light at the end of the tunnel may not be as far off as I imagine.

From Dr. Brittani James's and Dr. Brandi Jackson's discussion on healing while being black and in medicine, to Dr. Mark Shapiro's continued advocacy as an ally and his ability to utilize and recognize his privilege to uplift women in medicine—the 2021 Women in Medicine Summit was filled with pivotal information to catalyze the change necessary to combat the inequitable gender gap within our medical healthcare system.

Hearing stories from the women in medicine who paved the way for my success inspires me to work hard and to make the necessary connections to be the change I hope to see in medicine. It is evident that not all women have the privilege of breaking glass ceilings; it is for this exact reason that we must continue to thrive and strive to uplift one another as we rise. Disparities of race, social class, ethnicity, age, and religion continue to pollute the system we trust to care for us. What better way to capitalize on these stereotypes than to utilize them to our advantage while simultaneously dismantling the system?

Chapter 4: *Community*

In his excerpt from "Horae Canonicae," W.H. Auden mentions the passion in the eyes of men who do what they love. The annual WIM Summit posits this fact to be especially true of women in medicine whose drive for gender equity and patient care fuels their vocations on a daily basis.

"You need not see what someone is doing
*to know if it is **her** vocation,*
*you have only to watch **her** eyes:*
a cook mixing a sauce, a surgeon
making a primary incision,
a clerk completing a bill of lading,
wear the same rapt expression,
forgetting themselves in a function.
How beautiful it is,
that eye-on-the-object look."
—W.H. AUDEN, "HORAE CANONICAE"

Social Media as a Key to Connection*

Mya L. Roberson, PhD

I often hear, "Hey, I know you from Twitter!" as I turn on my heels to identify the source. A variation of this exclamation has become commonplace at scientific conferences.

Particularly in a time characterized by so much distance, the use of social media can be helpful for connecting new areas of scholarship, fellow scientists, and the people most affected by the work we do.

As a cancer care delivery scientist, I find social media to be an invaluable source of information and connection with people living with cancer. Many patient-led organizations curate incredible content that those of us connected to oncology can read and engage with. The substantial social media presence of patient-led organizations enables us to maintain a pulse on issues that matter to people living with cancer.

For me, social media connections with patient advocates have even led to patient-partnered research projects. Through social media, I could form connections with people I may have never encountered otherwise. These outlets provide an opportunity to expand who we know and to remain grounded in what matters.

Beyond connection with people affected by cancer, social media also provides us with a unique opportunity to share our science. What better way to test our communication skills than to distill our main messages into 280 characters—including spaces! The inherent word limits of apps like Twitter force us to be as concise and clear as possible when communicating important messages.

It also provides us an opportunity to spread our work beyond our peers to the broader public. Public science communication is an important way to democratize knowledge around cancer that can often remain in ivory towers. Often, our peer-reviewed articles are hidden behind paywalls that are not always accessible to broad populations. By tweeting out the main messages of our work, we exponentially expand the number of people it potentially reaches. In an era where well-vetted information can be hard for the average person to discern, thoughtful public-facing communication from oncology professionals becomes even more important.

Beyond public communication, social media potentially provides us, as professional women, the opportunity to get our work seen by our peers as we frequently lack visibility through traditional channels. Research by Luc and colleagues has shown that articles shared on Twitter often have higher citation counts than those not disseminated broadly.[33] Putting some thought into how we communicate our work beyond the peer-reviewed publication is one small way to increase the visibility of the great work being conducted by women.

---

33 Luc, Jessica GY. "Does Tweeting Improve Citations? One-Year Results From the TSSMN Prospective Randomized Trial." Annals of Thoracic Surgery. vol. 111, no. 1, Jan 2021, pp 296-300. doi: 10.1016/j.athoracsur.2020.04.065.

Using social media in a professional capacity has a wide array of benefits for oncology professionals. In a time when many of our major gatherings have gone hybrid or remote, it provides an opportunity to find and stay connected with both our peers and the people affected by cancer.

* This piece comes from the partnership between the WIMS Blog and the Healio Women in Oncology blog:
Roberson, ML. Women in Oncology (blog): Social media is a key to connection. Healio, June 7, 2022. Available at: https://www.wimedicine.org/blog/social-media-as-a-key-to-connection. Reprinted with permission from Healio.

Through the Eyes of a Woman Physician from Across the World: The Internet's Evolution as a Forum for Support and its Continuing Promise

Pallavi Rohela, MBBS, MPH

The service shuttle picked up speed on the empty road at night. The Midwestern town where we were interviewing had arranged for transportation back to the hotel after the pre-interview dinner. I got talking to my co-interviewee. She was a fellow South Asian, albeit of Pakistani heritage, and had grown up in the United States. We talked about our families.

"My mom was a doctor in Pakistan. When she came here after marriage, she did all the USMLEs. But it did not work out that time," she trailed off. As often happens in such situations, her mother became a full-time mom to raise her children, all of whom grew up to either work in healthcare or were studying towards becoming healthcare professionals.

That residency interview season was my fourth year after graduating from medical school in India, and the last year that I would make the filter of the five-year graduation cutoff date for most programs. I went unmatched. In the days that followed Match Day, I often revisited the years that had gone by.

I recalled losing the spot in my preferred medical school by one rank and going to another over a thousand miles away from home, right out of high school. I recalled the sheer dismay I felt when the promise of internet connectivity, thought to be an equalizer of knowledge and opportunity access, was crushed by the old government-built hostel (dormitory) attached to my medical school. The hostel lacked drinking water supply on all floors, let alone cable or internet connection. I recalled the trips I made to the nearby internet café, which charged exorbitantly for 15 minutes of internet access. I recalled learning about the USMLE exams during hospital electives in the United States on a social media platform called Orkut. I felt awe when I first entered the well-equipped examination rooms in the Midwestern University Hospital where I rotated. I remembered every positive evaluation from attendings I worked with, in different settings, and the hope it gave me to keep working towards a residency training spot.

I also reflected on how the right opportunities became scarcer, as my sole source of information—the internet—reached saturation. On anonymous internet forums, the follow-through of posts and genuine, insightful discussions were not regular or amenable to future referrals. The emails I received about the ECFMG-International Advisors Network did not specifically talk about mentorship and sponsorship and it seemed more focused on providing a platform to publicize alternative career choices without sufficient context. The American physicians I had worked with did not know how exactly they could help me—a non-US International Medical Graduate—reach the next stage in my career.

Realization dawned that in absence of a large alumni network and personal contacts, all of my networking efforts would continue to be futile. My engineer spouse, his extended family of engineers, and their circle of engineer friends offered some advice, but the gulf between the nature of medicine and engineering professions left me wanting more meaningful career assistance. Further, concerns about the ticking biological clock crept in. I faced a mix of bafflement from some quarters at worrying about having a child "so young," and questions from others at not having had a child yet!

The year I was pregnant, I focused solely on my health for multiple reasons. I experienced severe judgment about my choice and heard more expressed worries about the "gap in the CV" than congratulatory statements. Career anxiety enveloped my pregnancy. In moments of solitude at night, I wondered if my story, too, would turn out to be one of sacrifice—like my former co-interviewee's mom.

So far, I had been following the commonly known route: study, pass the USMLEs, find electives and observerships, get recommendation letters, and apply through ERAS. What does one do after going unmatched if a return to the home country is not feasible? While I was aware of nonmedical career paths I could take, I was struck by the limited information about how individuals made those choices, how fulfilled they were, or if they saw potential for continuing growth in those paths. There was no single, credible forum where people shared their journeys. There was no research on the unique challenges faced by women physicians who were non-US

IMGs who had limited insider contacts. There was no avenue to find collaboration opportunities where non-US IMG women could be matched by skill sets to willing mentors who understood their backgrounds and challenges. Women in my situation not only need career support, but they also need life advice, because starting over in a new country and raising a child with limited community involvement is difficult.

Over the years, Orkut disappeared. Facebook fell in and out of favor. Twitter emerged as an excellent vehicle for forging connections and brewing engaging conversations with individuals who are real and traceable. After a long lull, the internet was again opening possibilities for me. It was on Twitter that I first found out about the advocacy work done by the Women in Medicine Summit. I started to see how lack of timely career guidance and reproductive freedoms impacted career paths for women physicians globally. It is my sincere hope that the Women in Medicine Summit forum, too, will embrace the global community of women physicians *as well as* women like me—physicians from foreign shores who come to the United States in pursuit of their American Dream.

The author acknowledges Dr. Devika Das for her inspiration and role modeling.

An Alternate Point of View from a Social Media Introvert

Amna Anees, MD, FACP

I still remember that day when my existence came into question. After presenting a talk at a national forum, I was attending the rest of the conference. This was during the COVID-19 pandemic, so the conference was virtual. I read in the comments a reference to the Twitter handle for a speaker and decided to log on to my Twitter account. I had made that account about five to six years back during an AAIM chief resident meeting where there was a workshop on social media and how to use Twitter effectively. I have to be honest here, I forgot all about it afterwards until I dusted off my app, found my password somewhere in the deep dark vaults of my phone, and logged on to Twitter on the day of my conference. There was so much appreciation for all the talks and speakers on Twitter for that particular conference. However, I didn't see any mention of my name or my talk. It was almost as if my talk did not exist. Looking back, other than the obvious possibility that my talk was a horrible one (entirely possible), the other possibility was that I did not exist on Twitter and I had not associated my speaker profile with a Twitter handle. Okay no worries, I thought. But like any human being, I felt a bit down that this was truly representing the phenomenon "out of sight, out of mind." Basically, if it is not on social media, it did not happen! This made me wonder, would I get more speaking opportunities?

Going forward, I noticed that for talks at different conferences, there was always appreciation for folks who were active on Twitter but less for those who are not on Twitter. While this may seem appropriate (for the lack of a better word) to some, it irritated me initially. Does this mean that people who are not active on social media are less academically robust or poor presenters? No. I also noticed that with #medtwitter and the Match, there were a lot of potential candidates posting about themselves on Twitter. This raised a question in my mind: Is there any way this is introducing a potential bias? Are applicants who are active on social media and able to interact more with programs more likely to be "known" to the program? Is this more important when everything has gone virtual with COVID? Does this lead to a form of selection bias where candidates who are not on social media due to lack of resources or interest are selected against? While I agree that social media is the way forward, I want to highlight that people who are not on social media can also be academically robust. Applicants who are not posting actively on Twitter can also be very promising candidates. When we give shout-outs on social media, it should not matter if the person is on social media or not. Inclusion should always be practiced. Not everyone has a "spentor" (a combination of sponsor and mentor). Not everyone feels comfortable with self-promotion, however gentle it may be. This should not mean that their talks or work should not be highlighted. This can also have an impact on further career growth.

I am truly curious about how one keeps bias out of the selection of a speaker or a candidate, for example, if one knows them better just from a social media outlet. This also makes me wonder about our "algorithmic" feeds and whether they further introduce bias and do not allow us to see the other side of the picture? While this may not have mattered ten years ago, it certainly does seem to matter now when there is so much polarity to everything. I do not have answers to these questions but I do wonder about the direction in which we are headed.

This is truly an era where the world is a global village. The ability to make connections and friends now is so exciting but while we reach for the skies, I just wonder if we are leaving behind some people unknowingly and unfairly. Where is the balance and how do we decide it? After all, it is a question of existence for some.

Building a Sense of Community through Digital Scholarship

Gabriela Azevedo Sansoni

For those who are not familiar with the term "digital scholarship," a very Wikipedian definition is "the use of digital evidence, methods of inquiry, research, publication and preservation to achieve scholarly and research goals."

It is not uncommon to have co-authors meet on social media, especially Facebook groups for professional researchers. There are also survey researchers with entire protocols written around sharing the questionnaire via social media or even the direct use of metadata to determine risks of getting a certain disease based on your location.[34]

The number of peer-review publications grows every day, written by the very same group members on the use of social media, hashtags, and engagement among healthcare professionals. These nontraditional, facilitated paths into academia for aspiring

34 Fan, Chao et al. "Effects of population co-location reduction on cross-county transmission risk of COVID-19 in the United States." Applied Network Science. vol. 6, no. 1, 2021, pp. 14. doi: 10.1007/s41109-021-00361-y

physician-researchers are also a new niche of study for already reputable academics.

More than a few of these studies highlight the importance of networking, mentorship, and advocacy for gender equity in medicine and surgery. A nonexhaustive list of some examples that caught my attention in the past few months is found below.

- "Women in Cardiology: Role of Social Media in Advocacy."[35]
- "Social Media as a Means of Networking and Mentorship: Role for Women in Cardiothoracic Surgery."[36]
- "Social Media in the Mentorship and Networking of Physicians: Important Role for Women in Surgical Specialties."[37]
- "Women in Radiology: Creating a Global Mentorship Network through Social Media."[38]
- "Social Media and Gender Equity in Oncology."[39]

In addition to publication output, these endeavors have also created communities. Even if I am not active on social media, I still try to find space online to engage and contribute to creating communities in academia and medicine.

35 Patel, Hena and Annabelle Santos Volgman. "Women in Cardiology: Role of Social Media in Advocacy." *Current Cardiology Reviews*. vol. 17, no. 2, 2021, pp 144-149. doi: 10.2174 /1573403X16666200203104851

36 Luc, Jessica G.Y. et al. "Social Media as a Means of Networking and Mentorship: Role for Women in Cardiothoracic Surgery." Seminars in Thoracic and Cardiovascular Surgery. vol. 30, no. 4, 2018, pp. 487-495. doi: 10.1053/j.semtcvs.2018.07.015

37 Luc, Jessica G.Y. et al. "Social media in the mentorship and networking of physicians: Important role for women in surgical specialties." *The American Journal of Surgery*. vol. 215, no. 4, April 2018, pp. 752-760. doi: 10.1016/j.amjsurg.2018.02.011.

38 Retrouvey, Michelle et al. "Women in Radiology: Creating a Global Mentorship Network Through Social Media." *Journal of the American College of Radiology*. vol. 15, no. 1 Pt B, January 2018, pp. 229-232. doi: 10.1016/j.jacr.2017.09.029.

39 Knoll, Miriam A and Reshma Jagsi. "Social Media and Gender Equity in Oncology." *JAMA Oncology*. vol. 5, no. 1, January 2019, pp. 15-16. doi: 10.1001/jamaoncol.2018.4647.

A large community with many specialty groups is *Cochrane* (www.cochrane.org). You might have heard of it as it is quite big in systematic research. On the *Cochrane* platform, there is point-based membership. You need to accumulate points to be a member. There are no options of paying a fee or using your credentials to automatically become a member. The only other ways of becoming a member is working for them or having an "outstanding contribution to *Cochrane* over many years." There is a portal called TaskExchange where individuals can sign up for tasks and post tasks for others to fulfill. The gamification of the process makes it fun and rewarding to contribute to real science.

There are different ways of contributing to *Cochrane*. For example, you can contribute to expert opinions and consumer input, translate articles, join reviews, etc. In order to provide consumer input, you are usually required to be a patient yourself or to have a personal relationship with someone who is a patient. More obviously, expert tasks require expertise and translation requires language knowledge. Note that not all tasks posted are for *Cochrane Reviews*, and some are just from individual researchers looking for collaboration.

Despite my somewhat limited medical student skill set, I was able to connect with scholars and researchers and contribute to science. I was a consumer reviewer once. The process was very straightforward and efficient and happened through a survey. In addition, I usually volunteer to translate articles in Portuguese and Italian to English. My favorite experience, however, was when I was able to translate a Dutch article from the 1960s to English. Dutch is my fourth language so I was already excited about this challenge. What made it more interesting was seeing how academic writing was different back then. There wasn't such a rigid structure and citing other articles sounded more like mentioning friends who ran similar experiments in neighboring countries.

Another nice initiative I came across just after joining *Cochrane* was EvidenceAid (www.evidenceaid.org). EvidenceAid aims to bring the general public closer to evidence-based information contained in (most of the time) systematic reviews via short communications and summaries of the studies, available for free. They have collections on different topics (e.g. earthquakes, COVID-19, Zika, Health Systems Resilience, etc.) and are currently working on having it all translated into many different languages. Much of the work is done via volunteers and interns. I recently signed up to join their small team that is updating the Malnutrition Collection and I am currently navigating how it works.

So, if you are not a fan of social media, like me, or if you just want an extra layer of privacy, you can still benefit from the amazing perks of Digital Scholarship—networking, creative projects, and scholarly output, and community!

On Writing as a Woman in Medicine

Jennifer Caputo-Seidler, MD

The overarching theme of the 2021 WIM Summit was "The Power of Stories." Keynote speaker Dr. Kimberly Manning taught us to embrace the legacy narrative. Dr. Jessi Gold and Dr. Arghavan Salles showed us how to use writing as a tool for advocacy. Dr. Brittani James and Dr. Brandi Jackson gave us goosebumps with their use of storytelling in "Healing While Black." As an aspiring woman physician writer, here are some of my key takeaways from the 2021 WIM Summit.

Practice deliberately.

As clinical trainees, we learn to distinguish normal breath sounds from the rhonchi of pneumonia or the crackles of heart failure by listening to many lungs, presenting our exam to our attending teachers, and receiving feedback on our findings. It is only through practicing the physical exam with direct feedback that we become expert clinicians. To become better writers, we must engage in this same rigorous deliberate practice. We must write and receive feedback on our work. Both Dr. Kimberly Manning and Dr. Suzanne Koven spoke of how they used blogs as a space to engage in this writing practice. A blog not only allows you to write in the creation of posts, but readers can also give feedback through comments or the contact page. This feedback will help you as a writer understand what resonates with your readers. Over time you will develop the topics and style of writing that lands best with your intended audience.

Write first, then find the platform.

Even if your ultimate goal is a publication, the first step should be the writing itself. Write the story you are obsessed with, the one you are curious about, or one you feel others need to hear. After you complete the piece, figure out the best fit for that piece to submit for publication. You may be surprised at where your work ultimately ends up. Dr. Suzanne Koven shared a piece she wrote that was ultimately picked up by NPR, an outlet that wasn't on her radar when she wrote the essay. Writing with only one publication platform in mind may prematurely limit your publication options.

Put it on your CV.

Dr. Avital O'Glasser led a breakout session on reclaiming the CV. She is at the forefront of a movement to have the CV represent more than just peer-reviewed publications. Humanities scholarship through narrative writing and writing for advocacy definitely belongs on your CV. Because much of this writing is disseminated in the digital space, you can and should hyperlink the piece. Don't forget to share your work's impact by citing the number of views on a blog platform or the number of impressions on social media!

Writing is a powerful tool for sharing our experiences and expertise as women in medicine. To harness that power, writing needs to be a priority. With competing demands for our time and attention, writing won't happen unless we are purposeful about making time for it. Block time on your calendar to dedicate to writing. Don't let the fear of failing to generate Pulitzer-worthy prose keep you from starting. Recognize that writing is a skill that can be honed with practice. And, remember that improving your craft requires feedback. If you don't have a personal contact who can serve as a writing mentor, a blog is a great starting place to get your writing out there and see what resonates. If you don't want the upkeep of maintaining your own blog, consider digital publication spaces, like those available through the Women in Medicine Summit, where you can receive feedback on your writing from experienced editors and have your work shared broadly with others in medicine.

SECTION TWO

"The Work"

The work—the work we do, the work we TRY to do despite what holds us back, and the work we need done for us and with us to further gender equity efforts. We start this section fresh off pieces about the role and critical importance of community (Chapter 4) and dive into the data that exists regarding gender inequity and gender bias (Chapter 5). We then harness momentum to reinvigorate discussions about professional development and exciting, intriguing, and energizing opportunities for personal and professional growth (Chapter 6), especially through the lens of mentorship and sponsorship (Chapter 7). Finally, we look at how HeForShe support is a critically important facet of these discussions (Chapter 8).

Chapter 5

GENDER INEQUITY

We Need to Talk about Bruno. Signed, Cassandra

Eve Bloomgarden, MD, and
Avital O'Glasser, MD, FACP, SFHM, DFPM

October of 2021, WIMS published "Call Me Cassandra" on their blog, which drew analogies between the ancient Greek character and healthcare workers during the pandemic.

Cassandra was a Trojan princess and priestess of Apollo. She was gifted with the ability to utter true prophecies but then cursed to never be believed. Her resulting treatment was awful and dehumanizing: depending on the telling of the myth, she is viewed as a liar, an idiot, or mentally ill.

Healthcare professionals have been battling both COVID-19 and misinformation for more than two years. And in that time, we've gone from being called heroes, to being ignored, to being yelled and screamed at for continuing to advocate for masks, vaccines, and physical distancing. We've been trolled, doxxed, targeted, and harassed. Since the beginning of the Omicron surge in late 2021, we know many HCWs who have expressed renewed feelings of being Cassandras.

We are Cassandras.

But, are we also Brunos?

And who *IS* Bruno?

"WE DON'T TALK ABOUT BRUNO!"[40]

For those who have not yet watched the new Disney movie *Encanto*, we won't spoil the story. Briefly, Bruno is the black sheep of a large family whose members are blessed by "the Miracle" with individual powers. Bruno was gifted with the ability to prophesy the future, which is not well received by his family and community as they are "left ... grappling with prophecies they couldn't understand."

Ultimately, confusion and disappointment in the prophecies gives way to significant fear and stigma towards Bruno. His family misunderstands Bruno's role in creating the future by thinking "Your fate is sealed when your prophecy is read." However, Bruno doesn't choose future events—he reports what has been shown to him. He gets blamed nonetheless.

Like Cassandra, Bruno's gift from the Miracle ultimately becomes his curse: and he is shunned, ostracized, ignored, and humiliated for trying to keep his family and friends safe from harm. Unlike Bruno, we can't help but wonder about the degree to which gender bias led Cassandra to be so easily dismissed. Is it knowing the future that we fear, or is it the messenger *woman*?

Cassandra was gaslighted. Bruno was canceled. Are we destined for the same fate as pariahs, social outcasts who are "always talking about the virus"? And what does this mean for society, if the truth is so fervently denied? Do we succumb to misinformation, let the wool cover our collective eyes, and take the easy path? The very idea is anathema to healthcare workers, and yet here we are, years into the pandemic.

---

40 Miranda, Lin-Manuel. "We Don't Talk About Bruno". *Encanto.* 2021.

Bruno and his challenges, like many of the characters in *Encanto*, have been embraced by healthcare professionals.[41] Like Bruno, our advocacy has not only fallen on nonlistening ears, but it has been thrown back in our faces in ways that contribute to burnout and moral injury. And, we are blamed for things that are clearly not our fault—like the Omicron surge.

Do we wait for a miracle? Can we afford to wait for a miracle? Do we hope that somewhere there is a Mirabel who will save us? Or do we cave to *mundus velt decipi* and our desire to be deceived? Does the world want to know the truth? Or, as painful as the truth can be, is it easier to cancel it while relegating us to behind the walls of the hospital while ignoring the elephant in the room.

Is that the point where we are? We don't talk about Bruno ... or COVID-19?

Fortunately for Bruno, his niece Mirabel powers through the loud cries to ignore Bruno and not talk about him: "I really need to know about Bruno; gimme the truth and the whole truth, Bruno."[42] By facing a truth that others did not want to hear, Mirabel champions the family's ultimate safety and wellness.

According to the myths, Cassandra is ultimately deemed worthy of her dedication. In *Encanto*, Bruno is ultimately welcomed back to the familia with loving arms. To our fellow Cassandras AND Brunos—we HEAR you. We SEE you. We BELIEVE you. Keep advocating and warning. We will continue to talk about you and the important messages you are spreading.

So, if you're willing to talk about Bruno, please DM ...

---

41 Lycette JL. "Under the Surface, a Reflection on the Movie *Encanto*." Medscape, 11 Jan. 2022, https://www.medscape.com/viewarticle/966009#vp_2.
42 *Encanto*. Directed by Byron Howard and Jared Bush, Walt Disney Studios Motion Pictures, 2021.

A Randomized Controlled Trial, N=2

Tanya M. Wildes, MD, MSCI

For twenty years, I have been living in a randomized controlled trial (RCT) with a sample size of two.

The independent variable by which my co-participant and I were randomized in the mid-1970s is the presence of a second X chromosome vs. the privilege of a Y chromosome. The dependent variables observed have included both qualitative and quantitative measures related to being physicians in academic medicine, ranging from leadership opportunities to academic promotion to salary. The primary outcome we will examine today was the seminal time-to-event outcome of academic promotion, which was the first time I fully grasped the professional impact of our different treatment groups.

My husband—the co-participant—and I met as undergraduates when we were both pre-med. We happened to sit next to each other in a statistics class senior year. We joke that he asked me on a date with the dad joke forerunner, "What are the *odds* you'll go out with me?"

Fast forward a decade, with a wedding squeezed in at the beginning of our fourth year of medical school, we strode through our chosen residency and fellowships, with me pausing momentarily to give birth to our son at the end of fellowship. Then began our faculty journeys at the same institution. We worked hard, taking care of hundreds of patients, writing papers and grants, juggling shared calendars and nannies, and vying for book-reading time with our toddler.

Our paths differed somewhat, with mine more focused on research and his on institutional leadership and clinical program development. But we walked in parallel, both briefly instructors then moving up to assistant professors. The evident differences in our experiences, such as salary and leadership opportunities, seemed easily explained by our different chosen fields and focuses.

I never questioned that a meritocracy existed, having grown up hearing the praise of bootstraps and the payoffs of hard work. To me, it stood to reason that promotion would naturally follow if I worked as hard as I could for long enough. Then, there would come an "Atta, girl!" and promotion would follow.

In the fall of 2016, my husband came home and informed me that he was being recommended for promotion and that he was to submit his portfolio. I thought "Cool, must be time for that!" I assumed I would now be promoted in a similar timeframe: I had 3 times the number of publications as he did and had been awarded several grants. I do not present this data to suggest my CV was superior to his or to degrade his promotion; we simply had different career capital, and I had accumulated lots of what is typically valued as the currency of academic medicine.

So I entered my annual review meeting confident that I, too, would hear that I had "made it." I introduced the topic and was promptly shot down with "You're not ready . . ."

I inquired as to why and was told that maybe I would be . . . if I received a certain type of grant. I was baffled. I was being evaluated against criteria that were not actually written requirements.

On the outside, I kept myself steady, walking the ridiculous tightrope of a woman advocating for herself without being deemed "pushy." But, inside, I was decimated.

Everything I believed about achievement was collapsing. I numbly walked out of the office, the walls of everything I believed about merit crumbling around me. I couldn't reconcile it. I objectively met all the written, published criteria for promotion, so how was I "not ready?"

The pieces started to drop into place. I was experiencing gender bias. This leader had a picture in their mind about what an associate professor looked like, and I was not it. But what kind of RCT uses different measures for the same outcome?

I reformatted my CV. I started with the promotion criteria and pasted my activities and accomplishments under the criteria each fulfilled. This did get the process moving forward and I was eventually promoted two years after my husband's promotion. However, this delay will continue to follow me for my career. Some institutions require or at least consider a certain number of years at current rank before promotion to the next rank. He will likely become a full professor before I do. With salary often tied to rank, I may ultimately make less money over my career than if I had been promoted alongside my peers when I initially met criteria.

There are some limitations in interpretation of the primary outcome in this small RCT. Our appointments were in different academic departments, which may have different conventions and processes for proposing candidates for promotion. However, both are governed by the same written criteria. The use of unwritten rules allows unconscious bias to flourish and contributes to disparities in promotion. And though I report here on only one small trial, my experience is not unique.

My experiences were similar to those detailed in a recent qualitative study published by Murphy et al. of the experiences of women faculty in academic medicine.[43] In an analysis of almost 600,000 medical school graduates from the late 1970s to the 2010s, using time-to-event analyses, women physicians were 24% less likely to be promoted from assistant to associate professor. The trend did not improve over time.[44]

Another limitation of this study is that I am non-Hispanic white; I grieve that faculty members of color face even greater barriers. A recent study of Association of American Medical Colleges data through 2019 demonstrated that faculty members who are of a minority race/ethnicity underrepresented in medicine (URM) continue to experience lower rates of promotion from the assistant to associate professor level compared to their white and Asian counterparts.[45]

43 Murphy, Marie et al. "Women's Experiences of Promotion and Tenure in Academic Medicine and Potential Implications for Gender Disparities in Career Advancement: A Qualitative Analysis." JAMA Network Open. vol. 4, no. 9, September 2021, pp. e2125843. doi: 10.1001/jamanetworkopen.2021.25843.

44 Richter, Kimber P. et al. "Women Physicians and Promotion in Academic Medicine." *New England Journal of Medicine.* vol. 383, no. 22, November 2020, pp. 2148-2157. doi: 10.1056/NEJMsa1916935

45 Xierali, Imam M. et al. "Recent Trends in Faculty Promotion in U.S. Medical Schools: Implications for Recruitment, Retention, and Diversity and Inclusion." *Academic Medicine.* vol. 96, no. 10, October 2021, pp. 1441-1448. doi: 10.1097/ACM.0000000000004188.

My awakening to the fallacy of meritocracies was an earth-quake in my life. I underwent a massive shift in what drove me each day. While I had always been passionate about my area of research, I no longer worked with a dual purpose of advancing my career while advancing science. I had seen behind the curtain and knew that the academic treadmill did not have a finish line. There was no "arrived." Achievements are not what would make me "enough." Author David Brooks calls this first path of achievement *The First Mountain*.[46] This RCT outcome helped move me onto the Second Mountain, one focused on contribution rather than achievement. I was still passionate about the science but also focused on making sure others didn't suffer the same decimation I did.

This experience also impacted my family. My husband has become a committed #HeforShe. And that little boy born at the start of our faculty journey? He's been watching too. And he is one amazing little budding feminist, willing to speak up when he sees injustice or lack of awareness of issues related to gender bias. In fact, a recent lunchroom conversation gave him the opportunity to help a middle school classmate understand the differences between sexual assault, sexual harassment, and gender bias.

Twenty-five years ago in a stats class, sitting beside a person who would become my life partner and co-participant in this RCT, I learned that scientific questions are framed with null and alternative hypotheses. My experience has led me to reject two interrelated null hypotheses: that a meritocracy exists in academic medicine and that academic promotion was not influenced by gender. I look forward to the day where we will reject the alternative hypothe-

---

46 Brooks, David. *The Second Mountain: The Quest for a Moral Life*. First edition. Random House, 2019.

ses, when the risk of bias in subjective evaluation of "readiness" is recognized, systems are put in place to minimize this risk, and each faculty member's qualifications for promotion are evaluated equitably.

In this essay, I conflate sex and gender for narrative purposes.

Women in Surgery

Anuja Dattatray Mali

"There is no limit to what we,
as women, can accomplish."

—MICHELLE OBAMA

History of women in surgery began over one hundred fifty years ago when a young woman diagnosed with uterine cancer confided in her friend, Elizabeth, that she would have been spared her worst suffering if her physician had been a woman. This testament led Elizabeth to study medicine, thus starting a revolution. Dr. Elizabeth Blackwell, the very first reported woman to graduate from medical school in 1849 and pursue a career in surgery paved the way for women to practice medicine independently. Yet, surgical fields still seem to be dominated by men. This begs the question: Why does this still hold true today?

In North America, a survey of surgeons carried out at the recent turn of the century showed only 20.3% of surgeons were female.[47] In fact, less than half of all the residents in surgical spe-

---

47 Gargiulo, Debra A. et al. "Women in Surgery Do we really Understand the Deterrents?" *Archives of Surgery.* vol. 144, no. 4, 2006, pp. 405-407. doi: 10.1001/archsurg.141.4.405.

cialties are women. Women have made significant contributions to the field of surgery throughout history, and the number of women entering the surgical field has significantly increased over the last few decades. Despite the increased ratio between female and male medical students, men still significantly outnumber women in a number of specialties, most notably in surgery. Currently over half of the medical students are women but less than half are applying to surgery. Surgery has traditionally been considered a very male-dominated specialty in spite of the increasing number of women who are graduating from different medical schools.

Many times, female surgeons are frequently asked why they chose to be surgeons. In my opinion, women are attracted to surgical careers for reasons similar to that of their male colleagues. I think it is not about becoming a surgeon, it is the prestige that comes with being a surgeon.

In 2005, in an invited editorial describing her experience as a woman in surgery, Jo Buyske, MD, wrote, "Most women surgeons in my era, and certainly those before, have spent our careers being as sexually invisible as possible while attending to the business of learning and practicing surgery. The goal was to be accepted as a surgeon, not a woman surgeon."

Why are there so few women in surgery?

An article in the *International Journal of Surgery Global Health* noted that women can be subjected to gendered expectations about work-life balance and steered away from a career that could take time away from starting families and raising children.[48] However, lifestyle is not only a women's issue. In surgery, many of these

48 de Costa, Josephine et al. "Women in surgery: challenges and opportunities." *International Journal of Surgery: Global Health.* vol. 1, no. 1, July 2018, p. e02, doi: 10.1097/GH9.0000000000000002

issues have been identified as pushing women away from engaging surgical practice. These include the perceptions that the quality of life amongst surgeons does not fit the burden of caregiving possibilities that women bear. Furthermore, surgical training programs are themselves considered to be demanding and competitive. For women who struggle with gendered perceptions of what women can and cannot do, this presents yet another barrier in pursuing a career in surgery. As a result, women are subject to a hidden higher standard to enter and thrive in the surgical field, despite the fact that research shows that "female doctors perform equally as well as their male peers on measures of medical knowledge, communication skills, professionalism, technical skills, practiced-based learning, and clinical judgment."[49]

And even more troubling is that more women are leaving medicine due to lack of flexibility, fewer opportunities, and less support. With the increasing number of women entering medicine but the stagnant number of women entering surgical practice, there is a clear signal for change. Change is needed because allowing women in surgery to continue to experience the impact of gender bias is completely unfair and simply unacceptable. We can change that. Women belong everywhere in society and especially in healthcare, as female physicians have been linked to improved patient outcomes.[50]

---

49 Seebacher N. Gender equity in medical specialties: Level Medicine Inc. Summer Research Fellowship Report, 2016. Available at: http://levelmedicine.org.au/resources/completed-fellowship-papers/gender-equity-in-medicalspecialties/. Accessed April 25, 2018.
Referring to Thomas W. Teaching and assessing surgical competence. Ann R Coll Surg Engl 2006;88:429–32 and Pico K, et al. Do men outperform women during orthopaedic residency training? Clin Orthop Relat Res 2010;468:1804–8.
50 Tsugawa, Yusuke et al. "Comparison of Hospital Mortality and Readmission Rates for Medicare Patients Treated by Male vs Female Physicians." *JAMA Internal Medicine*. vol. 177, no. 2, February 2018, pp. 206-213. doi:10.1001/jamainternmed.2016.7875

Let's make surgery a better profession not just for women but for everyone seeking to provide health care in an environment free from discrimination. We can change the system if only we are brave enough to stand up to it.

"Don't let anybody tell you that being a woman or wanting to have a family or anything is a barrier. It's not the easiest thing in the world to do, but it's possible."— Dr. Bonne, MD[51]

---

51 Haskins, Julie. "Where are All the Women in Surgery?" AAMCNews. 15 July 2019, https://www.aamc.org/news-insights/where-are-all-women-surgery.

Two Women in Oncology Break Barriers in Male-Dominated Genitourinary Oncology Field*

Alice Yu, MD; Monica Chatwal, MD

It's easy to see genitourinary oncology as a man's world.

Many cancers that genitourinary oncologists treat affect only men, such as prostate, testicular, and penile cancers. Although bladder and kidney cancers can affect everyone, they are more commonly diagnosed in men. Unsurprisingly, the physicians who treat these diseases reflect that patient pool—they're mostly men.

According to data from the 2021 American Urological Association Census, only 10.9% of all practicing urologists in the US are women.[52] Although that number has increased from 7.7% in 2014, growth of women in the field compared with growth in the number of urologists overall is decreasing.

---

52 American Urological Association. The State of Urology Workforce and Practice in the United States. American Urological Association, 22 April 2022, https://www.auanet.org/documents/research/census/2021%20Census%20Report.pdf

Opening the Field

At Moffitt Cancer Center, we are the only two women in a group of thirteen physicians in the genitourinary oncology department.

We are focused on opening new opportunities for patients and offering different perspectives when it comes to care. We are also committed to seeing the field open up to more women providers.

In our experience, most patients don't view us differently from our male colleagues. However, there are rare incidents where patients have asked to see a male provider instead.

Overall, having two women in the department creates more opportunities and choices for our female patients, and we have even had male patients ask to transfer to us because they prefer a woman's communication style and demeanor.

Still, there are times when gender discrimination makes the job harder, especially in our training. It's no secret that female residents are treated differently by nurses and staff. Our judgment and authority are questioned a lot more than those of a male colleague. If a male attending is straightforward when giving an order, no one questions it. If a woman has that personality, she is often labeled as difficult. The simple action of a patient calling us by our first name can also hit a nerve. It's essentially a matter of respect, and we don't think it happens as often to our male colleagues.

Thanks to the strong leadership and positive culture at Moffitt Cancer Center and its genitourinary oncology department, we both have only ever felt included and supported by our male colleagues here. In order for things to change in the field as a whole, though, genitourinary oncology needs more female physicians and leaders.

Importance of Mentorship

Although the number of women in the genitourinary oncology field is growing, it's growing too slowly and could take decades for the number of women to equal the number of men.

Mentorship is an essential part of this change. Mentors can encourage fellows to see the field and consider it a promising career path without feeling uncomfortable or ostracized in the male-dominated environment.

As female genitourinary oncologists, we are working to increase our presence across the country.

The Society of Women in Urology and the Women in Urologic Oncology groups continue to grow and have done tremendous work promoting female urologists in academia. American Society of Clinical Oncology (ASCO) has a dedicated space with various organized events for women during the annual meeting, including mentoring sessions, and they have a Women in Oncology blog published in ASCO Connections.

For our numbers to grow, though, culture must change.

We need to continue to talk about these issues and promote introspection so people can recognize their bias toward physicians who are women. It won't be easy, but we won't give up hope. We want to one day close the gender gap, one female urologist at a time.

* This piece comes from the partnership between the WIMS Blog and the Healio Women in Oncology blog:
Yu A, Chatwal M. Women in Oncology (blog): Two women in oncology break barriers in male-dominated genitourinary oncology. Available at: https://www.wimedicine.org/blog/two-women-in-genitourinary-oncology. Reprinted with permission from Healio.

Let's Get Loud

Darilyn Moyer, MD, MACP, FRCP, FIDSA, FAMWA, FEFIM

Let's get loud—because the ones we need cannot become what they cannot see.

The imperative has never been greater, the data never more compelling, and the solutions never more daunting. As Covid-19 descended on our population, it amplified the deep and dark underbelly of health inequities and systemic racism by exacerbating the unacceptable status quo. How and why must all the stakeholders in healthcare work together with our patients and communities to correct these inequities for our patients and healthcare workforce?

The data for patient-physician racial and gender congruity leading to improved patient outcomes is accumulating. Nonetheless, there has not been a proportional increase in Black men entering medical school since 1978. Despite the rapid, recent expansion of new medical schools and medical school classes, none of the last thirty have been in conjunction with a historically black college or university (HBCU).

Despite more than thirty years of organizations trying to move the needle to ensure that women and others underrepresented in medicine (URiM) have their proportional representation in chair and impactful dean positions, the needle has barely moved. We should not suffer the tyranny of low expectations of just getting one woman and/or URiM to a position of power. We need tectonic shifts that give appropriate representation proportional to patient populations. In 2015, 51%, 17.6%, 13.3%, and 1.2% of the US population were women, Latina/o, Black, and American Indian, respectively.[53]

The tsunami of data regarding systemic disadvantages and barriers to women and others underrepresented in the healthcare workforce is incontrovertible. Now is the time to fix this, as potential new physicians and others in healthcare cannot be what they cannot see. As the world's largest medical specialty organization, with 160,000 members,[54] the American College of Physicians (ACP) has a strong voice in representing internal medicine physicians. Working towards health justice, becoming an anti-racist organization, and achieving a diverse, equitable, and inclusive healthcare environment are part of ACP's strategic priorities and current goals.

As I stated in an interview for the WIM Conference:

"Every society should do the foundational work of systematically and comprehensively resetting its organizational vision, mission, and goals through a lens of justice, equity, diversity, and inclusion. This foundational work should be directly accountable to the fiduciary board and governance body, and should permeate every structure in the organization including committees, councils, and local chapters.

---

53 Age and Sex Composition in the United States: 2015. United States Census Bureau. Available at: https://www.census.gov/data/tables/2015/demo/age-and-sex/2015-age-sex-composition.html
54 https://www.acponline.org/about-acp/who-we-are

These new structures, informed by metrics, need to be transparent, evaluated, adjusted, and continuously measured. Societies need to generously share their data through publications and presentations. There is excellent language in medical school, graduate medical programs, and healthcare environment accreditation and regulatory standards that recognize that more just, diverse, equitable, and inclusive (JEDI) healthcare environments lead to safer and higher quality outcomes for our patients. The Council of Medical Specialty Societies (CMSS), composed of 45 national physician professional societies representing > 800K physicians, has DEI as one of its top 2 strategic priorities.

In healthcare and life, we need to walk the talk. It's time to communicate, collaborate, and execute a plan to get our healthcare system to a more JEDI place. And while we're on this journey, let's make a difference for those who previously couldn't see what they could be.

Let's get loud!

The Gender Wage Gap Is Not New, but Negotiating for What's Important Can Help*

Anees B. Chagpar, MD

Significant disparities exist in pay, promotion, and perquisites between the sexes in every field, not just in medicine, and this has been the case for centuries.

It's unfair and it's not right, but sadly that knowledge alone is not sufficient to change the status quo. Simply pointing out the disparities is very much analogous to the experiment in which Capuchin monkeys who, seeing their counterparts get grapes (the preferred payment for doing a task), throw the less favored cucumber back to investigators and rattle their cages. We can rail against the inequities, but what we truly need is a strategy to affect action.

So how do we do that? Some have advocated for greater transparency as a means to correct disparities. Certainly, some have found that transparent-structured compensation plans may reduce, but not eliminate, wage disparities. Others, however, have found that transparency alone does not mitigate inequities and may, in fact, exacerbate the feelings of discrimination that exist in the workplace.

As the COVID-19 pandemic taught us, it's not all about the money. A recent report in the *Harvard Business Review* noted that more women physicians are either thinking of cutting back their clinical practice or leaving the workforce all together.[55] Sure, pay inequities have something to do with that, but it's also a reflection of some employers' lack of flexibility for maternity leave, provision of child and elder care, and the myriad of other things that leave women feeling—to a greater degree than men—burned out and undervalued.

Although having programs that provide for paid leave, onsite day care facilities and flexibility in call schedules can help, it's important to realize that these efforts will be more important to some women than to others. Indeed, there may not be a "one-size-fits-all" approach to ensuring women feel valued in the workplace.

What might be more effective—both for reducing pay inequities as well as for ensuring women feel valued—is if women simply negotiated for what was important to them. It is well known that "women don't ask," and that we tend not to advocate as strongly or as well for ourselves as we do for others. As such, some have advocated for negotiation training as one means to help reduce the inequities that exist. I know what you're thinking: One more thing, as though women don't have enough on their plate! And why should the onus be on women? These are fair points; however, in order to recognize the diversity within each gender, and the individual values each of us has, it behooves us to know how to negotiate effectively without being perceived as being overly demanding, greedy, belligerent, or worse.

55 Dudley, Jessica et al. "Why So Many Women Physicians are Quitting." *Harvard Business Review.* 19 Jan. 2022, https://hbr.org/2022/01/why-so-many-women-physicians-are-quitting

Many institutions and professional groups, including the Association of American Colleges, have included negotiation training in their leadership workshops—particularly for women. I have taught many of them over the last decade. They are, in general, universally well received as fun, energizing, and motivating, but one wonders whether they truly make an impact. During the pandemic, when in-person workshops ceased to exist, the American Medical Association put out a call for applications for the Joan Giambalvo Award for the advancement of women. I was honored to receive that award and set about not only to create a virtual negotiations workshop but also to test its efficacy. To my complete surprise, our virtual negotiation training workshop resulted not only in improved knowledge and confidence in negotiation skills, but further actually resulted in improved outcomes! Women stated their knowledge and confidence in negotiation as a result of the workshop and three months later, 40.7% of respondents stated they had used what they had learned: 57.7% had negotiated for pay, 41.7% for a promotion and 32% for job-related perks. These negotiations went "better than expected" in 26.6%, 30% and 37.5% of instances, respectively. Before the course, only three (2.9%) felt that their last negotiation went "very well" or better; three months after the course, 28% felt their last negotiation after the course went "very well" or "extremely well" ($P = .002$). To achieve such statistically significant results with a relatively small sample size blew my mind!

To be clear, closing the gender gap will require a multipronged approach, and I have no delusions that this will be easy or fast. But knowing that we can start to turn the flywheel by honing negotiation skills gives me optimism for the future.

* *This piece comes from the partnership between the WIMS Blog and the Healio Women in Oncology blog:*

Chagpar AB. Women in Oncology (blog): The gender wage gap is not new, but negotiating for what's important can help. Healio, April 8, 2022. Available at:

https://www.wimedicine.org/blog/the-gender-wage-gap-is-not-new-but-negotiating-for-whats-important-can-help. Reprinted with permission from Healio.

Chapter 6
PROFESSIONAL DEVELOPMENT

Using the Professional Curriculum Vitae to Tackle Pandemic-Related Inequities

Avital O'Glasser, MD, FACP, SFHM, DFPM, Shikha Jain, MD, FACP, and Vineet Arora, MD, MAPP

The COVID-19 pandemic has permanently altered the healthcare landscape and created unimaginable challenges. It has directly threatened the physical safety, as well as mental and emotional safety, of healthcare workers. It has dramatically reshaped how physicians work, utilize their time outside of work, educate their children, and care for their families while keeping them safe. And as the pandemic persisted, so did exhaustion, burnout, and ongoing disruptions to careers and personal lives.

Many physicians work in academic centers, with expectations for annual productivity—frequently, though not exclusively, scholarly productivity including publications, research, and presentations at medical conferences and other academic institutions—in addition to direct patient care responsibilities. Some institutions implement "promotion deadline decisions," sometimes also known as "up or out" structures that require benchmarks to be met within a certain number of years of employment as a condition for retainment. Additionally, our colleagues outside of traditional academic medicine may strive for scholarly productivity or other professional development goals.

These criteria can be challenging to meet most years and the COVID-19 pandemic added significant stress to these preexisting pressures. Within the work environment, physicians were deployed to inpatient services during surges, outpatient practices had to rapidly transition to telehealth, and new leadership and advocacy roles required time and attention. Outside of the immediate work environment, childcare challenges including rapid shifts to home-schooling diverted time and energy away from academic bandwidth.

The pandemic has negatively affected working mothers, including women physicians more than men by, for example, leading to a decrease in publications, more at-home responsibilities, and home-schooling responsibilities. Women remain disproportionately affected by its economic impact and burden on personal responsibilities. The preexisting "mommy tax," the "minority tax,"[56] and the "second pandemic"[57] of structural racism have only been compounded.

In the early spring months of the pandemic, our group (including two male allies) recognized that it was more critical than ever to ensure that pivots, novel work, and other academic disruptions be captured on the professional CV. We created the "COVID-19 Curriculum Vitae Matrix".[58]

---

56 Rodríguez, Jose E et al. "Addressing disparities in academic medicine: what of the minority tax?." *BMC Medical Education*. vol. 15, no. 6, 2015, doi: 10.1186/s12909-015-0290-9

57 Manning, Kimberly D. "When Grief and Crises Intersect: Perspectives of a Black Physician in the Time of Two Pandemics." *Journal of Hospital Medicine*. vol. 15, no. 9, September 2020, pp. 566-567. doi: 10.12788/jhm.3481

58 Arora, Vineet M et al. "Covid19 Contributions On A Professional CV." Explore the Space, LLC, June 2020, https://www.explorethespaceshow.com/white_papers/covid19-contributions-on-a-professional-cv/.

The matrix includes multiple categories of contributions, helping the user articulate both ADDED efforts in response to the COVID-19 pandemic and lost/modified professional opportunities:

- Direct clinical contributions
- Research
- Education
- Service and volunteerism
- Advocacy
- Social Media

Women in medicine are uniquely threatened by the COVID-19 pandemic, which promised to stall and even set back progress towards gender equity. A "she-cession" in academic medicine would lead to "a lost generation of women falling off the path," reducing work hours, or leaving medicine altogether.

For decades, publication volume and subsequent number of citations have been the currency of promotion and tenure pathways in academia. Prior to the pandemic, there were signs that alternative and nontraditional promotion benchmarks were being considered and debated.[59] We hope that this matrix spurs additional conversation about what defines meaningful and impactful contributions within medicine. While we developed the matrix to support gender equity in medicine, we hope that all colleagues will benefit from the open-minded conversations it generates. But the work will still require several discussions. For example, just last month, a new publication revealed women's CVs were rated lower than men's CVs even when they were identical.[60]

59 Mullangi, Samyukta et al. "Is it Time to Reimagine Academic Promotion and Tenure?" *JAMA Health Forum.* vol. 1, no. 2, 2020, pp. e200164. doi:10.1001/jamahealthforum.2020.0164

60 Franco, Marina C. et al. "The impact of gender on researchers' assessment: A randomized controlled trial." *Journal of Clinical Epidemiology.* vol. 138, October 2021, pp. 95-101. doi: 10.1016/j.jclinepi.2021.05.026

When the time comes, we cannot move past the COVID-19 pandemic and return to "prior state." Amidst the suffering and struggles, we must harness the innovations, pivots, and lessons learned. We hope that a new recognition of the need to broaden the definition of what "counts" in academic and nonacademic medicine, along with a means to articulate that, is a lasting outcome of academic medicine's response to the pandemic.

A CV of Failures: Dissolving the Illusion of Perfection

Jillian Bybee, MD

If the five-year-old me who first dreamed of being a pediatrician could see me now, she would be in awe that we made it. She did not truly know if it was possible. If the twenty-eight-year-old me who dreamed of becoming a pediatric intensivist could see me now, she would let out a sigh of relief; the upcoming years of achievement and delayed gratification were "worth it." As the present me, a pediatric intensivist medical educator, I appear to have reached all the goals that I have set for myself so far but I know something that the past-me did not anticipate: I have failed during each phase of my career in order to get to where I am.

As a recovering perfectionist, it still makes me squeamish to write the word fail, let alone associate it with myself. For most of my life, I took great care to be sure that I did not fail. Or, if I did, I made sure to never disclose my failures publicly to comply with familial and societal expectations. I used a smoke-and-mirrors approach of hiding my shortcomings to convey perfection.

I am not the only woman in medicine who has done this. As women, we have been conditioned to make things look "effortless."

If we are struggling, we learn we should hide it from the world to continue the charade and not be a burden to others. "Never let them see you sweat."

I bought into this approach earlier in my life and career, and I racked up the achievements necessary to secure a place in pediatric critical care medicine. But the process almost broke me, resulting in a major depressive episode and burnout during fellowship. Unfortunately, it has broken many of our female physician colleagues who have taken their own lives or chosen to leave medicine. And countless others are currently struggling.

Though there are numerous unique drivers of burnout, mental illness, and attrition, for me, other-oriented perfectionism fueled by imposter phenomenon was close to the top. I carefully curated my outward appearance and achievements to stand out while also fitting into academic culture. Thus, it was paramount that I keep my insecurities and failures hidden. I succeeded for a long time until I was no longer able to do so.

In academics, we have an entire document dedicated to what we have achieved: the Curriculum Vitae (CV). It highlights where we have gone to school, awards we have received, positions we have held, grants we have secured, etc. What gets left out are all the things that have not gone to plan: positions not obtained, research not published, institutions not attended, and so forth. In each of these areas, I have failed to achieve something that I attempted, but that is not reflected on paper.

The message transmitted by the achievements on someone's CV may be misconstrued by others who are struggling to achieve their own goals. We may perceive that the person with a long list of achievements on her CV has never experienced struggle or failure, especially if we have never heard that person disclose their hardships.

To shine a light on the illusion of perfection in academics and to break down the shame often associated with being imperfect, Melanie Stefan introduced the "CV of Failures" in *Nature* in 2010.[61] In this piece, she recommended keeping a running list of the failures you have had: unsuccessful applications, refused grant proposals, etc. By doing so, she argued, we remind ourselves and others that succeeding takes the ability to recover from failure rather than being able to avoid failure completely. Subsequently, others have made their CV of Failures public, further normalizing the process of failing forward.

I now understand that to be human and to try is to invite failure. Having survived failing greatly on occasion in my own life and having heard many others whom I admire admit their own failures, I have been able to shed the shame that previously accompanied my own imperfection. Through failure, we learn how to carry on, to start again, or to pivot. Failures are part of being human because we are all works in progress.

As a leader in medical education, I now find it particularly important to share my past and present failures with the trainees and the early career faculty members around me. The earlier we are in our life or career, the less experience we have with navigating failures and coming out on the other side. This, coupled with the illusion that everyone we admire is "perfect" can contribute to burnout, as I experienced earlier in my career.

Learning to fail forward and allow imperfection in myself has been transformational. Embracing the vulnerability of failing and disclosing my failures to others has not resulted in them finding

61 Stefan, M. A CV of failures. *Nature* 468, 467 (2010). https://doi.org/10.1038/nj7322-467a

me less competent. But it has allowed me to build stronger relationships with those around me. Additionally, I have become more likely to take professional risks, embrace my own creativity, and find more joy in my personal and professional life.

If you are struggling to maintain the illusion of perfection that so many of us women in medicine try to uphold, perhaps it's time to let it go, embrace your CV of failures, and repeat the words of Samuel Beckett:[62]

> *Ever tried.*
> *Ever failed.*
> *No matter.*
> *Try again.*
> *Fail again.*
> *Fail better.*

---

62 Becket, S. "Worstward Ho". Grove Press. 1983.

Pivoting Isn't Quitting

Kelly Cawcutt, MD, MS

No one likes a quitter.

Quit—to leave a place permanently; to get rid of

Pivot—the central point something spins on; to turn in any direction

For the longest time, I felt that quitting and pivoting were the same. And I am NOT a quitter.

In medicine and in my career, though, this has meant the path I started down was straight and narrow and I did not waver from the mapped course. Sure, there could be obstacles thrown down my path forcing me to traverse the flood or even surmount the unexpected mountain. But the way was set.

The path was clearly mapped out full of academic and clinical research, research mentors, a master's degree in clinical and translational science, and a long list of publications paved that intended trajectory to continue down that classic academic road.

But in my heart of hearts I knew that this journey was laid out for me by a different mapmaker and was not truly a path entirely of my own choosing. I felt as lost as a seafarer on a starless night, a victim of the waves, who lacked both the conviction and dedication to stay on course. This was the beginning of the end, where I simultaneously started to wonder if I still loved medicine and felt increasing burnout due to lack of joy in my day-to-day work.

And it hurt. I felt like a failure. I felt like I had wasted years. I felt the guilt of wanting to carve out an entirely new path. I felt like a quitter and I hated myself for it. But I knew (and know) that my heart has always been in business and leadership—aka often referred to as the dark side of medicine; the enemy camp: health care administration (*audible gasp from the audience*). Yes, we desperately need more physician leaders in administration. I love the strategizing that comes with trying to impact health care at the organizational level. This is the path I am drawn to follow. I recognize that not everyone will understand or be supportive, and that is normal and ok. As long as I enjoy the work, feel that I am creating a positive impact, and I am true to my authentic self, that is what matters. I did not learn this easily or quickly.

Here are some of the hard-earned truths I discovered:

- Changing courses may seem like quitting at first, to both you and to others. For those who cannot understand and who continue to believe it is quitting, or worse "selling out," know that they are not your people. Those are the mapmakers so stuck in their perceptions of what is, that they miss the adventure of the unknown and what could be.

- Quitting and pivoting may seem like semantics for some, but in truth the essence of their definitions clearly demonstrates that they are very different. I am not permanently getting rid of my career aspirations or medicine, but I (me, the person) am the center of my career, not research or academics or education, which means I am the central point that can spin and decide to turn in any direction. I can pivot, adjust my sails, and chart a new course of my choosing.

- Sometimes, the new course is indeed an adventure into the unknown, often requiring more courage than quitting. In that sense of adventure and its need of courage, we must remember that the unknown can be more beautiful than we could have imagined.

- Choosing to pivot is not what changes you—*you* change and thus you pivot. I wish I realized changing the mental construct to pivoting would empower and free me from the guilt and feeling like I was failing.

- Finally, it is still ok to truly quit something. You can make that choice. Do not ever let someone else tell you something different.

Top Pivot Tips:
1. Get your mindset straight. It is still ok to quit something. It is also ok to pivot. Everything changes, therefore, new career trajectories are a normal and an expected part of change. Accept that.
2. Decide if it is a quit or a pivot and then define AND own the why behind that. Be able to stand tall and be proud in that decision.
3. Have your pivot elevator speech prepared for those few who truly need to hear it (bosses, colleagues you may no

longer work with as often, etc.).

4. Lean in with curiosity, not judgment, when you or others around you change their trajectory. Be the supporter you would want for yourself. It will pay dividends back to you on the support you receive back.

5. Be kind, be humble, be honest, and strive to do it all with grace—for yourself and for those around you.

Our professional and personal lives have twists and turns. Changes in trajectories and career plans are going to happen. Change was hard for me but changing my mindset from "quitting" to "pivoting" was crucial. Hopefully, this wisdom and these tips provide you the psychological safety to pivot—not quit—on your own journeys.

Using Existing Citizenship Duties to Create Career Acceleration for Each Other

Eileen Barrett, MD, MPH

Employment-related citizenship tasks in medicine are widespread, necessary for operations, and often unfunded and undervalued. They are also often disproportionately performed by women,[63] and can contribute to a gender tax,[64] as well as a version of the majority subsidy.[65] Until we can transform our institutions to value, to compensate for, and to promote this essential work, some of it may be made more manageable by using it to promote others.

In my previous position, I was co-chair of our department's grand rounds planning committee and wrote about how this was used to advance other people's careers while improving peer education. On a smaller scale, I used a similar experience as director of

63 Guarino, Cassandra, and Victor M. H. Borden. "Faculty Service Loads and Gender: Are Women Taking Care of the Academic Family?" EconPapers, 28 June 2016, https://econpapers.repec.org/RePEc:iza:izadps:dp10010.

64 Armijo, Priscila R. et al. "Citizenship Tasks and Women Physicians: Additional Woman Tax in Academic Medicine?" *Journal of Women's Health* (Larchmt). vol. 30, no. 7, July 2021, pp. 935-943. doi: 10.1089/jwh.2020.8482.

65 Ziegelstein, Roy C and Deidra C. Crews. "The Majority Subsidy." *Annals of Internal Medicine*. vol. 171, no. 11, December 2019, pp. 845-846. doi: 10.7326/M19-1923

my division's monthly research presentation meeting to promote the great work of people often overlooked for speaking opportunities. Although coordinating this meeting fell under some of my compensated time in quality improvement, which is not the case for most in academia, it is still something many of us can do if we think creatively about our duties. In my case, this position had not been used to provide speaking and presentation opportunities particularly for women, early career faculty, and learners.

Over a two-year period, our once monthly hour-long research conference was transformed to highlight presenters who were women, students, residents, and early career professionals doing research projects in health equity. To maximize speaking opportunities and reduce the work of developing a presentation, two to three presenters were invited per one-hour session. Speakers with little presentation experience were provided draft slides that provided structure for presenting research and offered opportunities to have their slides reviewed ahead of time. In their speaker introductions, their expertise and achievements were highlighted and—particularly for students and residents—what an honor it was for faculty to learn from them. Afterward, presenters were provided a signed letter thanking them and highlighting their presentation. We encouraged presenters to share that letter with their faculty advisor (if still in training) or promotion dossier (if faculty).

How did it go? I don't know if the work was sustained after wrapping up my position, but it was personally so rewarding to receive feedback about how meaningful it was to have these opportunities available. We had 51 different scheduled presenters overall instead of the usual 24. Of those, 35 presenters were women some of whom presented multiple times, 10 were assistant professors, and 21 were students, residents, or fellows. The students in particular said it was their first speaking opportunity in front of faculty and that it was a confidence-building experience. Both residents and students said they would add it to their CVs when applying for their next steps.

This small redesign provided career acceleration for earlier career colleagues who are often overlooked for speaking opportunities, and I treasured seeing new presenters excel. Most valuable, though, was seeing how a group of talented, dedicated, and diverse presenters shared their innovative and unique research projects, often on topics that are incompletely covered in local research presentations, so that all of us could learn from them. I hope that their work is soon funded and valued as it should be in employment, leadership position selection, and promotion decisions. Until then, I hope more doctors replicate this small initiative in more workplaces and do it better. I look forward to hearing how that goes.

Empowering Yourself by Mastering the Stage: Tips to Being an Empowered Woman Speaker

Ankita Sagar, MD, FACP

Congratulations! You have booked your next presentation, workshop, or the main event—woman keynote speaker! At this time we know women are often not invited or paid to be keynote or conference speakers because of ongoing gender bias and suboptimal visibility for our content expertise. Your planning and efforts have yielded the opportunity to make your expertise renown as you continue to shatter glass ceilings.

Let's briefly review the steps that may help you go from good to great!

- **Ask questions of the organizers.** It is key to understand the objective of the meeting/conference. This is especially important if you are part of a panel or being interviewed. Ask for questions ahead of time, if possible.

- **Know your audience**. This cannot be overstated! Are they trainees, students, or faculty? Are executives or administrative leadership present? Ask your organizer if they can tell you about the audience members: number of attendees, roles, knowledge levels, preciding, or following presentations.

- **Be prepared, but don't memorize**. There is a fine balance between memorizing every word of every chart and rehearsing your speech material. Make sure you spend time on the material so you can refer back to it or guide your audience to the resources. Memorization takes away from your audience connecting with you. It is okay to sketch an outline or notecards, but avoid writing a speech.

- **Be a firework**. We hear the fireworks blasting off before we see them. And, then the colors and glitter leave us awestruck. Engage the audience members with your voice. Share the reason for your passion, expertise, or cause up front. You can open with a question, quote, or narrative.

- **Create a dialogue.** If you are presenting in person, avoid standing behind a podium and remember to move around and engage with your audience. If you are presenting virtually, look into the camera as you would when speaking with an ally or friend. Build in audience engagement, if possible. Some organizers have capabilities to use audience engagement tools such as polling, word clouds, chat features. If you are new to these tools, request a practice session ahead of time to work out any technical issues.

- **Choose high-quality visuals.** Always use high quality images, graphics, and charts. Do not use blurry images. Also, avoid an image that has a lot of text unless you are using it as a reference point to a simpler visual. Your audience may have difficulty following your path.
- **Avoid too much text.** Do not write out your content in full sentences. Use a format that brings *attention* to the most important points. Think of this as your attempt at highlighting 1-2 key takeaways per slide. You are not writing a paragraph or a book (*albeit, you may have the expertise to do so!*)
- **Time yourself.** There is nothing worse than the time running short. Audiences don't get to hear your phenomenal conclusion, organizers are stressed about running behind, and you are not given the opportunity to answer questions from the audience. Solution: time your presentation. You can even use PowerPoint to rehearse timings. If you are using a slide presentation, we recommend mapping out the time for yourself as below:
  » *Allotted time = 60 minutes*
  » *5 minutes for introduction*
  » *10 minutes for questions at the end (if any)*
  » *45 minutes for the actual content*
  » *At 2 minutes per slide, that would mean no more than 22 slides in your presentation.*
- **Remember to breathe.** Think of your presentation as a walk around your neighborhood with audience members as visitors. Don't rush through the topic. Take a moment to

pause, reflect, and connect to the theme of your talk. If you are on a panel or being interviewed, pause and restate the question to give you a few seconds to prepare.

- **Be enthusiastic.** If you are excited and enthusiastic about your topic, it will naturally come across to your audience. They will be more likely to enjoy the content even if it is about your pet cat. The more enthusiasm and excitement you have, the more likely you will be to land more speaking engagements.

- **Keep time for a conclusion**. Dedicating 3-5 minutes to your conclusion helps the audience remember why they are listening to you. Use this time to do a gentle recap and focus on what is next for them. Perhaps leave them with a future narrative that contrasts the story you shared at the beginning.

Being a woman who is invited to be a speaker is a step toward breaking down barriers and shattering glass ceilings. Congratulations on the opportunities you receive, and hopefully these tips help you thrive in these opportunities!

Leading as an Introvert

Purvi K. Shah, MD

Being an introvert is one of my defining characteristics. Those who know me well are aware that I will leave events when they get too "people-y." But more often I am not even present at such events. I need time to digest new information before I can form an opinion. I do not like conflict but I also don't like getting swept away in others' enthusiasm. I am, in a word, quiet.

When I was tapped for a leadership role at my organization earlier this year, I felt a small amount of pride and a significant amount of imposter syndrome, but primarily I felt exhausted in anticipation of the people-ing that this new role would entail. When I think of a leader, I think of someone who is an effortlessly eloquent speaker, someone who commands the room (physical or virtual), someone with palpable energy and excitement, and someone who can offer thoughtful reflection no matter the subject. In summary, NOT ME.

But I was chosen as a leader for a reason. So, over the past few months, I've been working on leading *as* an introvert instead of leading *despite* being one. Here's what I've found to be successful:

Know your strengths.

....

This was a theme at the recent WIM Summit. Dr. Kimberly Manning gave out an assignment to reflect on what we do well, what we are proud of, and what we've received positive feedback about. Laurie Baedke asked us to name, claim, and aim our super-powers. I am a highly effective communicator who is able to synthesize and articulate complex concepts. It was important for me to realize that this is a skill I have cultivated *as an introvert*! I argue that introversion itself is a strength and so does Susan Cain who wrote a book about it entitled *Quiet: The Power of Introverts in a World That Can't Stop Talking.*[66] Introverts are good listeners; they are thoughtful and reflective; they build connection through deep relationships; and, they are good at delegating especially when that involves delegating trust to others.

Get an external perspective.

....

I had the chance to participate in the absolutely transforma-tive WIM Leadership Accelerator over six months. Through its 360 evaluation and Hogan assessment, I learned a few things about myself. My introversion may come across as aloofness or dissat-isfaction; so now I work to include exclamation points in my com-munication! Under stress I may become irritable, stubborn, critical, and reluctant; I need to share this with the people I work with. My ideal work environment is one where I can concentrate and enjoy my quiet time, have structure and predictability, and don't have to compete for success. I know this isn't surprising but seeing it on

66 Cain, Susan. *Quiet*. Random House. 2012.

paper helped me realize that I can and should create this type of atmosphere for myself and my team. I also recognized that I need to continue to hone my communication strengths. I was prompted to complete a DiSC assessment after Stacy Wood's breakout session on communication styles at the WIM Summit. (The DiSC assessment measures four dimensions to identify one's communication style: Dominance, Influence, Steadiness, and Conscientiousness.)

Fake it 'til you make it.

I had about four weeks to transition into my leadership role. During that time, I studied the leaders that I admire. I tried to emulate what I appreciated about them and how I saw them sustaining engagement. For example, my boss does a great job of opening each meeting with an explanation of why we've come together, ends with a list of next steps, and asks if we need to get others involved; I have started doing this as well for the meetings that I run. For meetings that I attend as a participant, I review agendas and slides ahead of time and plan 1-2 points that I want to make; it is easier for me to speak up if I have already decided to do so. At the recent WIM Summit, I made it a goal to interact with people every day and specifically set out to compliment someone on her talk; this was all very uncomfortable but it was also profoundly rewarding. In the ultimate display of faking it, I gave a well-received talk at a national conference (and repeatedly questioned why I chose to do so until it was complete)! Feigned extroversion is a muscle. It needs regular exercise to get strong, becoming easier to use with practice; but, overworking it will cause damage.

Manage your energy.

....

I can tangibly feel my battery getting drained through increasing interactions with others. As a primary care physician, I had to quickly figure out how to manage my reserve in order to care for patients. I review charts ahead of appointments so that my time in the room is efficient but meaningful; this allows me to end appointments a few minutes early and retreat to my office to recharge. I have translated this into my administrative role as well. I am zealous about calendar management. If a day is filling up with back-to-back meetings, I put in holds for myself to take a break or tend to a task that is uniquely mine. If I feel myself getting sapped, I will turn off my camera for a meeting. I proactively let people know that in a difficult situation, I may not be able to come up with a plan right away but will ensure that we have follow-up scheduled. This allows me time to process in my own way without seeming flaky or indecisive. I tackle tasks in bite-sized pieces, especially those that may lead to more interaction. I have a hype song ("King of Anything" by Sara Bareilles) to get me ready for a challenging situation. And I have learned to say no! This is hard because I don't want to be seen as unreliable or not a team player, but I am working on a gut check to figure out if something is truly necessary for me to do. I embrace JOMO (Joy of Missing Out!) and don't worry about FOMO, not just in my personal life but at work as well.

I know it may seem strange for a self-professed introvert to be putting herself out there like this, but that's exactly why I wrote this piece. My introversion is an innate part of who I am and once I stopped seeing it as a weakness, I began to flourish.

Communication and Medicine—Lessons Learned at Johns Hopkins Bloomberg School of Public Health

Gabriela Azevedo Sansoni

Turn on the TV and switch to the news channel. Any day, anytime, anywhere in the world. Chances are there is either a pandemic, a medical emergency of the president or a celebrity, a generic scandal in hospital administration, or an ongoing vaccination campaign debate being broadcasted.

The status of being a student works as a protective shell as I currently have zero chances of being invited to give expert opinions on news broadcasts. As a curious person, however, I wondered with much interest on how it would feel to carry such privilege and responsibility of being a public health communicator. I confess I did not have to wonder for very long. And no, I was not invited to give an interview.

I was, instead, awarded a much more exciting opportunity. It involved twenty-four hours of master's level coursework spread over nine days, and it was worth it. The experience was possible thanks to a scholarship for the 17th Annual Johns Hopkins Fall Institute in Health Policy and Management and it was a wonderful course titled "Effective Presentations and News Media Interviews."

During the course, we had two main simulation exercises, both of which consisted of turning on the camera and microphone, smiling and speaking in a calm, clear manner, avoiding hand gestures and spinning on your desk chair, and looking trustworthy, serious, and yet amicable.

One of them was called a FlashTalk, or elevator pitch. You had to choose a topic that made sense to you, something that you did for work or school. At the time I chose to discuss my research internship work on cardiopulmonary exercise tests on Fontan circulation patients. I had a cohort of adults and children with and without Fontan circulation to study. Our test protocol was conducted on an ergometric bike with increasing resistance . . . and I could carry on for hours about this project. The truth is it is always going to be easier to talk about a topic you speak about frequently.

The second video was a live interview simulation. It lasted for seven minutes and had all the preparation a real interview would have. It was definitely interesting to try it out and I would say the simulation was very realistic. It gave me the chills and anxiety related to being live on TV. I made a fair amount of mistakes when it came to body language: chair spinning, looking down and to the sides, not looking directly at the camera, and so on.

Watching yourself on a recording can be a highly painful situation. It reminds you of how nonverbal cues are as important as verbal messaging. However, as we learned in class, doing good media interviews is just like any other skill. It can be learned. And as long as you remember the main messaging you're trying to get across, you can (try to) bypass some of the trickier questions by using tools like boomerangs and bridges (imagine re-bouncing a question or connecting a random answer to the main message you have to deliver).

I want to carry as much as possible from this course throughout my career. I had a great learning time in this short, intense experience. Being a public health communicator is more than being a good communicator or simply having an important, life-saving message to pass on. It is a healthy mix of both. It is having a duty—the duty of informing different stakeholders about relevant health related topics and official information, guidelines, and protocols to be followed. Sometimes they will be simple precautionary measures, others law-bound curfews, outwear (say masks, for example) and lockdowns. The course experience was paramount for me in getting to these conclusions and making me realize what being an effective public health communicator is as an individual and as a woman.

Reflecting on the #WIMStrongerTogether Chat

Michelle Brooks, MD, FACP

I raise up my voice—not so that I can shout,
but so that those without a voice can be heard . . .
We cannot all succeed when half of us are held back.

—MALALA YOUSAFZAI

The September 2021 Annual Women In Medicine Summit, which was held virtually because of the ongoing COVID-19 pandemic, kicked off with a Twitter chat in conjunction with the Society of Hospital Medicine. Forty-seven participants utilized the hashtag #WIMStrongerTogether to discuss topics surrounding the event's theme of finding the power of individual and collective voices. Within this theme, additional sub-themes emerged during the hour-long synchronous Twitter chat.

The first topic asked about barriers that prevent you from finding your voice or expressing yourself. Shared experiences included internal barriers such as fear, imposter syndrome, and ingrained cultural behavioral patterns as well as systemic barriers to equity, which prevent women from being recognized and rewarded for their work.

Within this segment of the discussion, a common theme was imposter syndrome, a psychological term that "refers to a pattern of behavior wherein people (even those with adequate external evidence of success) doubt their abilities and have a persistent fear of being exposed as fraud."[67] Many participants shared examples of subtle (and not-so-subtle) ways in which women are socialized to behave, recognizing that they worry about the way that they are being perceived and the repercussions of being authentic.

One thing that stood out to me is that several participants pointed out that women often receive mixed messages regarding their behavior at work, for example:

@WomenInPHM: *"I was told in a med school interview that I smile too much to be taken seriously as a doctor..."*[68]

@ShikhaJainMD: *"Then when you don't smile [people] ask why you aren't happy and that you should smile more."*[69]

I think about this in terms of the conflicting messages I have received as a woman in medicine: be confident but not overly confident; advocate for yourself but not too aggressively; be an excellent doctor but don't let it interfere with your home life; be candid but don't share how things *really* are.

Next, the discussion moved to the role of allies in amplifying and empowering voices. Allies are colleagues who are aware of the

---

67 Mullangi, Samyukta and Reshma Jagsi. "Imposter Syndrome: Treat the Cause, Not the Symptom." *JAMA.* vol. 302, no. 5, 2019, pp. 403-404. doi: 10.1001/jama.2019.9788

68 Women in PHM [@WomeninPHM]. "I Feel This in My Soul! I Was Told in a Med School Interview That I Smile Too Much to Be Taken Seriously as a Doctor. My Answer? 'I Won't Apologize for Being Happy to Be Finally Interviewing for My Dream Career." #Dropthemic #Wimstrongertogether." Twitter, 24 Sept. 2021, https://twitter.com/WomenInPHM/status/1441209191608246273?s=20.

69 Shikha Jain MD, FACP. [@ShikhaJainMD]. "Then When You Don't Smile PPL Ask Why You Aren't Happy and That You Should Smile More #Wimstrongertogether #Doublebind @Evebmd." Twitter, 24 Sept. 2021, https://twitter.com/ShikhaJainMD/status/1441209757029650432?s=20.

robust evidence on workforce gender disparities and who work to actively include qualified women through mentorship and sponsorship. Allies can speak up to prevent systemic and unsafe cultural barriers that restrain women from expressing their authentic voice. Emergent themes provoked by this question included amplification of women's voices, attribution for work, and intentional sponsorship. Using honorific plus last name rather than first name (ex. "Dr. Smith") can be a powerful way for allies to attribute ideas or focus attention back to the source of the idea. Women want to be in the "room where it happens." Because of imposter syndrome, we don't always feel like we have a voice at the table.

@ShikhaJainMD: I think @JulieSilverMD says it best. #quoteher #inviteher #sponsorher [70]

Several participants pointed toward the use of nontraditional platforms such as social media as ways for women to have access and voice.

@aoglasser: I have one word...wait for it...twitter. But in all seriousness—harness nontraditional means, including social media and 21ˢᵗ-century digital platforms to shake up the traditional amplification/spotlight pathways. [71]

The conversation then shifted to how the pandemic affected our abilities to find or use our voices. While virtual spaces have made it easier for some to find community, support, and opportunities, others pointed toward the inequitable impact of the pandemic on career productivity as a source of hardship/grief. The disruption of quarantines and loss of childcare were definite hardships.

---

70 Shikha Jain MD, FACP. [@ShikhaJainMD]. "I Think @JulieSilverMD Says It Best. #Quoteher #Inviteher #Sponsorher #Wimstrongertogether." Twitter, 24 Sept. 2021, https://twitter. com/ShikhaJainMD/status/1441210480895217671.
71 Avital Y. O'Glasser, MD FACP SFHM DFPM (she/her). [@aoglasser]. "#Wimstrongertogether I Have One Word..." Twitter, 24 Sept. 2021, https://twitter.com/aoglasser/status/1441210483298557958?s=20.

However, several participants in the chat felt that the pandemic opened avenues for their voice to be heard, especially through COVID-related advocacy and public education. Many participants were able to point to bright spots in the pandemic, including making connections and getting sponsored for more opportunities. There is potentially a disparity between those already in practice and those still in training, with those still in medical school or residency having difficulty ensuring adequate training and mentoring.

Finally, participants shared several important strategies for ensuring gender equity at the institutional and organizational level. Themes included intentionality in hiring a diverse workforce and ensuring fair distribution of types of work. Institutions can also support women in their workplaces with parental leave, and support for fertility, infertility, and adoption. Purposeful and meaningful changes in policy, guidelines, recruitment, and retention for women physicians is needed—with women invited to the table where these changes occur.

Through a moderated chat on social media about gender equity topics, participants were able to virtually connect with each other prior to the Women in Medicine Summit and identify shared experiences. Several of the topics were explored further during the conference sessions, and the discussion generated excitement for the content. For virtual conferences, an online chat allows for networking and connection to other attendees, and making for a great way to kick off the Summit!

MedLasso Presents: Ted Lasso, Gender Equity and Leadership

Eve Bloomgarden, MD;
Avital O'Glasser, MD, FACP, SFHM, DFPM

*Leadership: the ability to influence the group
toward an achievement of goals.*

As we celebrate Women's History Month and eagerly anticipate the 2023 premiere of the third and final season of *Ted Lasso,* it's time to acknowledge how this show has become a beacon of hope for the healthcare community. While it may seem like just another feel-good sports comedy on the surface, the magic of *Ted Lasso* is that the show is not really about football (soccer). The show's writing, direction, and choreography are brilliant and deliberately planned to convey subtle and authentic messages about psychological safety, allyship, and visibility.

In summer 2022, we joined Dr. Mark Shapiro's and Dr. Sayed Tabatabai's podcast on "MedLasso Presents: Ted Lasso, Gender Equity and Leadership" to explore leadership (especially women in leadership) and gender equity themes.[72] In honor of Women's History Month and the third and final season of the show, we have summarized our conversation.

This isn't a show only about football—far from it! The titular character, played by Jason Sudeikis, embodies communal characteristics that are typically associated with women, such as empathy, compassion, and vulnerability. Ted models masculinity without being misogynistic or hypersexual, and he treats women as equals without going out of his way to do so. He also role models team building, mentorship/sponsorship, and change management, which are essential tools for creating a level playing field for all genders.

But it's not just about Ted. The women on the show, played by talented actresses like Hannah Waddingham and Juno Temple, demonstrate the strength that can come from forming dyads and friendships. They are given and earn more leadership roles because of who they are and how they interact with others, not because of their gender. The women on the show aren't necessarily doing anything unique or different—what's different is the community and teams that surround them. These women are not raked across hot coals or shepherded away from or out of leadership roles. They earn and are given more leadership roles because of who they are and how they interact with others. (*"There's no Rebecca without Keeley!"*[73]). The show highlights the importance of diversity on a leadership team and gives credit where credit is due. Could the show actually represent the ideal working environment for women?

72 Bloomgarden, Eve and Avital Y. O'Glasser. Guest discussant. "Episode 291 : MedLasso Presents: Ted Lasso, Gender Equity and Leadership." Explore the Space Podcast. Explore the Space, 2022. https://www.explorethespaceshow.com/podcasting/medlasso-presents-ted-lasso-gender-equity-and-leadership/
73 Hannah Waddingham. Emmy Awards. September 2021.

Even the "one liners" and GIF-worthy quotes hold deeper meaning. "Women Up" is an invitation to allyship and sponsorship to get women a seat at the table. "Be curious, not judgmental" similarly energizes allyship and sponsorship—you have to be open to seeing something through a different perspective. Being curious is how you will succeed in inviting people who don't look like you to the table or giving them a voice. The allyship in the show is non-performative—and the show is not so much a "how to be an ally" lesson but a bigger, broader message of "what comes from successful allyship."

The show demonstrates so many high-quality leadership tools and techniques, especially for the equity space. This includes inclusive leadership, which is highlighted as a feature of leadership by women. It also highlights diversity on a leadership team. There are multiple examples of people NOT being gaslit—but instead credit given where credit is due. The show also models that healthy mentorship is bidirectional—there are skills needed to both be a mentor AND be a mentee.

So, let's continue to level the playing field (pun intended)—and stay tuned for Season 3 conversations!

Chapter 7

MENTORSHIP AND SPONSORSHIP

On Spentorship

Bethany Samuelson Bannow, MD, MCR

"Spentorship" is a fabulously descriptive term coined by Dr. Julie Silver to capture the concept that trainees, junior faculty, and even mid-career folks need not only mentorship but also sponsorship. In her fantastic discussions of the subject at the Harvard Women's Leadership Summit, she highlighted the fact that many female-identifying individuals, in particular, are "over-mentored but under-sponsored."

This concept recently became more salient to me during a discussion with a friend in a different specialty about a trainee. This trainee began a working relationship with their primary mentor who had a reputation as very successful and productive with those early in their training program. However, when the time came to discuss next steps in their career, this trainee found themselves struggling to get the advice and input they needed. Due to feeling hesitant to approach their mentor about anything other than their shared projects, the mentee was actively seeking advice from other faculty.

This situation got my friend and I talking about an important question: *what does mentorship mean?* Is mentorship really enough or should we in medicine be shifting our expectations to one of "spentorship," embodying both mentorship and sponsorship if we truly want to see trainees and junior faculty succeed?

Mentorship in and of itself is already an unfortunately vague term and varies enormously between institutions and individuals. Sponsorship, while a newer concept in medicine, is somewhat better defined. The technical definition of a sponsor is "one who assumes responsibility for some other person or thing."[74] In medicine, this effectively means "vouching" for, or expending networking or interpersonal capital on behalf of, someone junior. This can look like nominations for awards or promotions, recommendations for a role or responsibility that will result in career growth, or leveraging a network for additional support/resources.

To be clear, I am not advocating that every mentor needs to be a sponsor or a "spentor." There is both room and need for other kinds of mentorship, including project-specific mentorship, mentorship from those with shared experiences/identities (particularly true for those in minority groups, such as women of color, disabled persons, and the LGBTQ+ community) and short-term, defined mentorship through a society or training program. There is also room for those who may be primarily a sponsor and do less in terms of mentorship. However, most of us have one person we identify as our "primary" or global mentor in addition to seeking additional specific advice and input from others, and this is the role I wish to address.

In medicine, we talk a great deal about the importance of mentorship, having a mentor, being a mentor, and helping students, trainees, and junior faculty find a mentor. Institutions and societies

---

74 "Sponsor". Meriam Webster Dictionary. Available at: https://www.merriam-webster.com/dictionary/sponsor.

give mentorship awards to recognize those who, hopefully, excel at the art. Nonetheless, it is virtually impossible to find an agreed upon definition of good mentorship. And too often, especially for women, the next step—what a sponsor needs to do to get women seats at the table—is missing.

As scientists and physicians, we have a natural tendency to seek out objective criteria. In practice, this often means identifying those mentors with the traditional trappings of academic success, such as long lists of publications with mentees as first or middle authors. In this author's opinion, while important, publications are actually the lowest bar of mentorship. The next metric, which is perhaps slightly more comprehensive, is that of "success" in the mentee, meaning acceptance into a good/prestigious position, whether that be residency, fellowship or faculty role, or career productivity, such as receiving independent research funding. While this is typically a sign of more investment from a mentor, it may still be a better marker of the mentee's own persistence and skill. In the worst case, it could represent a mentee feeling forced down a pathway for which they may have skill but little passion.

Truly good mentorship, or spentorship, requires supporting and guiding a mentee down the best path for them. Sometimes this will lead to publications and accolades that reflect back on the mentor, but not always. It may involve facilitating mentorship relationships between a mentee and a different mentor when it becomes apparent that the mentee's interest diverges from the mentor's area of expertise. It may mean supporting a mentee in their need for work-life balance, even if this means a role outside of academics or a reduction in workload/hours. It may mean advocating for equity, fair treatment, or healthy boundaries, even when that involves facing backlash.

In short, spentorship comes down to a relationship between the primary mentor and mentee that extends beyond the project at hand. Like parenting, the goal must not be to produce a "mini-me" that practices and publishes just like the mentor. Nor must it be driven solely by the number of publications or presentations. The goal must be for the mentor to use their wisdom, experience and/ or network to help the mentee be the best version of themselves, whether that be in the clinic, in the lab, or in the classroom (or all three). Additionally, and perhaps most importantly, it requires clear communication and expectations about what roles the "spentor" can and can't fill and what needs the mentee has that may or may not be addressed within the relationship.

This communication is particularly important, as many trainees have little or no idea of what to expect or what they need from a mentor. Sadly, many careers have suffered from circumstances like those of the trainee described above, where a mentee envisions the primary mentor as someone who is actually only willing or able to provide project-specific mentorship and ultimately winds up without crucial guidance along the path.

"Spentorship" may or may not be for you but moving forward I exhort all of us to mentor when we can, sponsor when we can, and, most importantly, communicate clearly with those we advise.

One Small Grand Rounds Innovation to Increase Equity

Eileen Barrett, MD, MPH

The literature shows that most CME speakers are men—and that "manels" are still too common.[75] On CME planning committees, I have deliberately recommended speakers who were outstanding clinicians, great presenters, and as diverse as the audience. Often, the best presenters are those who have been overlooked due to implicit biases that we all have about who we perceive as experts and as leaders.[76,77] Several years ago, I helped start a Grand Round Steering Committee in the Department of Internal Medicine at the University of New Mexico to provide more flexibility, more relevance, and more equity. What we did is replicable to other places, and I hope others consider following suit—and doing even better.

75 Northcutt, Noelle et al. "SPEAKers at the National Society of Hospital Medicine Meeting: A Follow-UP Study of Gender Equity for Conference Speakers from 2015 to 2019. The SPEAK UP Study." *Journal of Hospital Medicine*. vol. 15, no. 4, April 2020, pp. 228-231. doi: 10.12788/jhm.3401.

76 Hall, William J. et al. "Implicit Racial/Ethnic Bias Among Health Care Professionals and Its Influence on Health Care Outcomes: A Systematic Review." *American Journal of Public Health*. vol. 105, no. 12, December 2015, e60-76. doi: 10.2105/AJPH.2015.302903

77 Mackenzie, Lori K and Shelley Correll. "Two Powerful Ways Managers Can Curb Implicit Biases." *Harvard Business Review*, 27 Aug. 2021, https://hbr.org/2018/10/two-powerful-ways-managers-can-curb-implicit-biases.

In once-monthly grand rounds slots, we introduced content outside of department subspecialties such as addiction, health policy, and leadership, as well as health equity, gender equity, and race and racism in healthcare and society. We invited experts from groups that are underrepresented as speakers, including minoritized people, trainees, and assistant professors. Through this deliberate approach, we achieved gender equity in presenters, had multiple assistant professors give grand rounds (which helped them in the promotions process), and had the highest representation of African American, Native American, Asian American, and Latinx presenters in the history of the Department.

Faculty and learners benefited from the content presented by diverse faculty and also benefited from seeing diverse presenters as leaders and role models for us all. When speakers better reflect the diversity of the community, it can increase feelings of belonging and possibly reduce imposter syndrome among trainees and faculty. It also positively affects the learning climate by showing that we value expertise and not solely years in practice—a measure that is often misunderstood as aptitude or excellence in presenting when selecting speakers.

A final innovation in grand rounds was creating the annual trainee research symposium, where trainees submit abstracts and receive mentorship on giving a great presentation. When trainees serve as grand rounds presenters, we are highlighting that trainee achievements are valued and that learning is bidirectional between faculty and trainees. Presenting at grand rounds also provides another achievement on their CV, and since our trainees are more diverse than at many other programs, the new opportunities to showcase their achievements was a form of equity and justice.

Like everything that we do, inviting speakers can provide recognition and validation of people who due to personal and group identities are less often offered professional advancement opportunities.[78] When we overlook diverse speakers, we miss out on their expertise and we risk perpetuating a glass ceiling and sticky floor that keeps minoritized people from the career recognition that is deserved. As you read about this one easy innovation, I'd like to ask you: What is *your* next step for supporting a peer or trainee in getting the professional recognition and career acceleration they deserve?

78 Yong, Ed. "Women Are Invited to Give Fewer Talks than Men at Top U.S. Universities." *The Atlantic*, 18 Dec. 2017, https://www.theatlantic.com/science/archive/2017/12/women-are-invited-to-give-fewer-talks-than-men-at-top-us-universities/548657/.

Chapter 8

HE/THEY FOR SHE

Are You Really a HeforShe Ally?

Eric Weng

If I had to make a disruptive prediction, I would say that men continually find themselves in disbelief when told that they aren't doing enough for HeforShe allies. I sat with my jaws touching the floor as I listened to Drs. Brad Johnson and David Smith present about male allies at the 2021 Women in Medicine Summit. As I listened, I began to ask myself, "How could I have been so oblivious?"

As an undergraduate student in the pursuit of eventually matriculating to medical school, I was honored to be able to join the room full of empowering physicians, PhDs, medical students of all years, and faculty during the annual "Women in Medicine Summit" held by founder and chair Dr. Shikha Jain. Across the board, from the main conference to break-off discussion sessions, nothing fell short of this year's title, "Evolution of Empowerment." In particular, I loved the presentation by Dr. Brad Johnson and Dr. David Smith. Dr. Johnson, PhD is a professor of psychology in the Department of Leadership, Ethics, and Law at the United States Naval Academy; Dr. Smith, PhD is an Associate Professor at the Johns Hopkins Carey

Business School. They co-authored the book, *Good Guys: How Men Can Be Better Allies for Women in the Workplace.*

Drs. Johnson and Smith began their presentation with eye-opening statistics showing how men and women are not on the same page in terms of allyship. Reported male involvement in gender diversity programs is at an all-time high,[79] yet if these numbers are accurate, the true question remains: Is that enough? And if so, why do we still have a persistent gender gap in health-care? More particularly, why do men continue to dominate leadership positions even though more women matriculate into medical school? [80]

Dr. Johnson states from Promundo/Equimundo's "So You Want to Be a Male Ally for Gender Equality?"[81] that, "77% of men agree that they are doing everything they can to advance gender equality while only 41% of women agree with this." He also states that "89% of men believe that they are good listeners to women reaching out about an experience of workplace harassment while only 58% of women agree to this." If indeed these numbers are to be believed, how do we translate an inherent desire to improve the system into actionable change with measurable solutions? How can we change the momentum of these equity movements into strategic, innovative change to finally close the gender gap in healthcare professions?

---

79 Boston Consulting Group. From Intention to Impact: Bridging Diversity in the Workplace. Boston Consulting Group, 2017, https://media-publications.bcg.com/BCG-Bridging-diversity-gap-workplace-Nov2017.pdf.

80 Person. "Men Dominate Physician Leadership. Here's One Way to Balance the Scales." Advisory Board, 6 Feb. 2020, https://www.advisory.com/daily-briefing/2020/02/06/national-female-physicians.

81 Equimundo. So, you want to be a male ally for gender equality?. Equimundo, 2019, https://www.equimundo.org/wp-content/uploads/2019/03/Male-Allyship-Study-Web.pdf.

We can start by asking why. Why is it that women account for the majority of medical school students but only make up 12% of medical school deans, 12% of department chairs, and 19% of full-time professors?[82] The answer lies in the lack of mentorship for women in medicine. Men often hold the positions of power in these systems. With that being said, men in these positions are more likely to be consistent with mentorship and sponsoring career-enhancing opportunities for men than for women.[83] However, possibilities for men to mentor and sponsor career-enhancing opportunities for women in healthcare are widely presented in meetings, projects, and everyday interactions. So why is it that men are not jumping at these opportunities? Dr. Johnson states in the research he did for *Athena Rising*[84] that the bottom line of men's hesitance stems from a battle of interpersonal allyship—a war rages with the stigma that has been created around the inability to collaborate with women unless in a romantic or sexual way. It also does not help that, in recent years, this has been exacerbated by confusion around the #MeToo movement. Men in positions of power may avoid working with women. They have become uncomfortable and fear giving women the wrong impression and ultimately facing the potential of sexual harassment or assault allegations.

I learned about several actionable changes that can be used to alleviate this problem. First, HeforShe allies should push back on these false narratives and reaffirm to everybody that these are not universal cases. Another possible option is to eliminate the nega-

---

82 Paturel, Amy. "Where Are All the Women Deans?" *AAMC*, 11 June 2019, https://www.aamc.org/news-insights/where-are-all-women-deans.

83 Anderson, Rania H. and David G. Smith. "What Men Can Do to Be Better Mentors and Sponsors to Women." *Harvard Business Review*, 17 Sept. 2021, https://hbr.org/2019/08/what-men-can-do-to-be-better-mentors-and-sponsors-to-women.

84 Johnson WB, Smith D. "Athena Rising: How and Why Men Should Mentor Women". *Bibliomotion*. 2016.

tive stigma around having men mentor and sponsor women in the workplace. Research shows that when men mentor and sponsor women in the workplace, they often help accelerate their course to success. Similarly, HeforShe allies should champion for women protégés in new roles and opportunities since this encourages other women to seek these same career advancements. As a result, this creates a more diverse workplace and improvements in team finances,[85] decision making,[86] and job satisfaction.[87]

Beyond the changes made at an interpersonal level, actionable changes in public allyship also need to be accomplished before systemic change to the gender gap can be made. Often, women are found to have less impactful voices in meetings and are thus more likely disregarded. Dr. Smith affirms that in the research he did for *Athena Rising*, women have stated that "they feel invisible in the workplace" or that "they feel like they have to work twice as hard." Furthermore, women are constantly faced with a descriptive and prescriptive bias.[88] When women lead in what is traditionally described as a "masculine way," they are labeled as bossy. And if they lead in a "feminine way," they are weak and unimpactful.

To tackle this conflict, having listening skills and developing empathy as to how women might be experiencing the workplace differently is very important. Furthermore, male allies making sure

85 Noland, Marcus et al. (February 2016). Is Gender Diversity Profitable? Evidence from a Global Survey. Peterson Institute for International Economics Working Paper No. 16-3, Available at SSRN: https://ssrn.com/abstract=2729348
86 Perryman, Alexa A et al. "Do Gender Differences Persist? An examination of gender diversity on firm performance, risk, and executive compensation." *Journal of Business Research*, vol. 69, no. 2, Dec 2015, pp. 579-586.
87 Pitts, David. "Diversity Management, Job Satisfaction, and Performance: Evidence from U.S. Federal Agencies." *Public Administration Review*. vol. 69, no. 2, 2009, pp. 328-338.
88 Heilman, Madeline E.. "Description and Prescription: How Gender Stereotypes Prevent Women's Ascent up the Organizational Ladder." *Journal of Social Issues*. vol. 57, no. 4, 2001, pp. 657-674.

that women's ideas are being heard and credibly received will aid in closing the gender gap. Additionally, taking the step to disrupt male colleagues when they make ill and unwanted comments lets women know that there are allies in the workplace. Saying things like "I did not find that funny" or "I do not like how you are treating women in this facility" can make a great impact. These disruptions bring attention and accountability towards unwanted comments and actions. These actions not only validate women's ideas in the workplace but also motivate other men in creating an alliable environment. Our desire to close the gender gap with actionable changes means understanding that these double standards need to be terminated.

The formula for closing the gender gap in the healthcare profession is clear. Now, more than ever, is the time to act—to educate your peers and colleagues about actionable changes. As previously stated, closing the gender gap not only creates a better environment but also benefits the business and the team in performance and success. I ask you to join hands with me in doing more than just the bare minimum in cultivating HeforShe allies and in advancing one step further in closing the gender gap in healthcare.

The Imposter Syndrome I Didn't Know I Had

Joseph Thomas, MD

Thanks to Twitter, I have learned from and been inspired by many women in healthcare, and I was excited to meet them in person when I attended the Women in Medicine Summit, engaging as a better HeForShe ally. In fact, I accompanied my favorite Woman In Medicine, my wife—Dr. Ashley Alex. That was fun, too. Between the two of us, I am the extrovert, but I knew I was a small fish in a big pond at the WIMSummit. I was excited to talk less and listen more.

In a hallway between breakout sessions, I found myself face to face with the one and only Dr. Shikha Jain. I geared up for my usual "Hi, I'm sorry to interrupt, but . . . " figuring she wouldn't have time to chat but I wanted to thank her for such a great conference. To my surprise, she spoke first.

Now, I am a cisgender, heterosexual, Indian-American man with the healthy ego that comes with that amount of privilege. I am a hospitalist, a few years out of training, with a passion for reproductive justice and, since about February 2020, combating medical disinformation online. I am comfortable in my current job and in my little corner of the Internet. But here, at my second-ever conference as an attendee, I found myself keeping fairly quiet, not always sure what to say. So, when Shikha said "Hi, I'm coming to meet you because . . . well, we should meet," I found myself reacting with thoughts I had not had in quite some time:

What? Why? I am just a schmuck.

Even Ashley, who has known me for a decade, when I relayed this story to her, pointed out that it was "weird to see this side of me."

Prior to the conference, we had dinner with one of my best friends who lives in Chicago and he asked if I thought my COVID education posts were actually making a difference. I pointed out that I'd received a message or two from folks who had changed their mind and gotten the vaccine. Ashley immediately chimed in with "and he gets questions every week from people about COVID and vaccines and other health issues."

I did not even realize how much I had downplayed my own impact. Ashley was not having that. When I later expressed to Shikha that I was not sure why she wanted to meet me, our conference chair/WIM president was not having that either. She pointed out some positive things she had seen from my social media presence and expressed happiness that I was present at the conference.

This is a terrible article for the Women in Medicine Summit book as I, a man, explain how two women made me feel better about myself. If anything, it was confirmation of what Drs. David Smith and Brad Johnson stated in their presentation about getting men to the gender equity table. Women have been doing this forever—encouraging each other through imposter syndrome moments and so many other things, to lift each other as they rise.

As a resident, I had not done well in seeking mentorship. I barked up the wrong tree with a couple of male attendings who were not interested in mentoring me, while there were female attendings who, in retrospect, were mentors/sponsors to me without my realization (not for their lack of trying). As Ted Lasso says, I needed to "woman up" long ago.

As I unpack my own mental barriers, I am inspired by the WIMSummit and the leaders I met. I have always found it easy to encourage others, but it's another step to recognize specific efforts and help others realize their imposter syndrome for what it is. It is my duty now to take those lessons back with me and make sure those I work with or train are made to feel the same way Shikha and Ashley made me feel. Two women helped me realize my own impact and, in doing so, inspired me to wield that power as a better ally.

The Bat and the Saguaro

Garrett S. Booth, MD, MS

The following is the acceptance speech by Dr. Garrett Booth upon receiving the #HeForShe #IStandWithHer Ally award at the 2022 Women in Medicine Summit.

Good afternoon, I wanted to first thank the organizing committee and the entirety of the Women in Medicine conference for such an amazing program.

As the recipient of the Ally in Medicine award, I can't help but think of a tree-based metaphor. Hear me out.

I'm not talking about the giant redwood who [*sic*] inhabits an amazing habitat full of environmental support, nourishment, work-life balance, equitable pay, and protection . . . What I'm thinking about when I hear the word "ally" is about a thousand miles to the south, in my home state, within the Sonoran Desert.

You see, in austere environments where there are limited resources, unrelenting environmental insults, and very minimal nourishment to grow and feed or sustain life of any form is where you really see allyships take place.

The Crown Jewel of the Sonoran Desert is unquestionably the saguaro cactus, capable of centuries of growth and development within some of the harshest conditions—no support, no nourishment, and relentless attacks from the environment. Despite all of these significant challenges, the saguaro cactus thrives. It stands tall despite all of the obstacles.

How does it do that? How is anything capable of thriving in such brutal conditions?

One such adaptation that the saguaro has embarked upon is to take advantage of the migratory interloper known as the lesser long-nosed bat. You see, this bat is an ally, but he didn't even know it, because he travels as a nocturnal animal feeding on the nectar of the saguaro blossom, inadvertently spreading its pollen from cactus to cactus, helping to ensure essential communication.

The lesser long-nosed bat had no idea that it was serving as an ally, this was all a byproduct of the evolutionary adaptations of the mighty saguaro. The bat just helped to facilitate the discussion.

This tiny two-ounce bat is what I think of when I think of being an ally.

I stand amongst the amazing, talented, diverse, hard-working, and inspiring saguaros of the healthcare world. And so, I accept this award with great humility and want to say thank you. Thank you to you all for letting this lesser long nosed bat help out in this journey. Thank you.

SECTION THREE

"The Change"

In this final section, we break down silos and explore how the change we need to implement is not only gender equity work. Concurrent with our gender equity advocacy, women are empowered voices for many other advocacy platforms. One could also argue that BECAUSE of the advocacy muscles we have built and strengthened through gender equity work, we are ideal advocates in other spaces. We embrace our strengths, skills, and passions to change the broader status quo—we are natural advocates but still need tools and resources to nurture the advocate identity (Chapter 9). Given the inordinate stressors of the last three years, which we know have disproportionately harmed women, we also share reflections and advocacy regarding the COVID-19 pandemic (Chapter 10). Because of its power, Chapter 10 also includes powerful pandemic reflections in the form of poetry. We then expand our lens to advocacy through anti-racism, anti-xenophobia, anti-transgender, and additional ways to help our communities (Chapter 11). Finally, we conclude this anthology with a discussion about abortion rights and women's health, especially as threats to these rights and access to care opportunities threaten us personally AND professionally (Chapter 12).

Chapter 9

ADVOCACY

Finding Agency Through Advocacy

Browning Haynes

The guilt and shame I felt watching a certain family's case spiral out of control has persisted to this day. The patient was an eight-year-old boy with a neurologic disorder and complex behavioral problems whose family had recently moved to Portland. Initially, my role was to help him and his family navigate the healthcare system as they began to establish medical care in Portland. However, it soon became clear that this family needed more than just navigation assistance, especially given the challenges brought on by the COVID-19 pandemic.

He and his family—which included his twin brother, parents, and extended relatives—lived in a two-bedroom apartment. Their housing was meant to be temporary while they searched for a more suitable place to live. I spent time with the family providing housing resources in addition to coordinating their medical care. But with the pandemic, his mother was laid off from work, and they could no longer afford a new home. A couple months later, I learned the entire family had developed chronic lung issues related to black mold in their apartment, which the landlord had previously been notified of but refused to remediate. I felt frustrated by the challenges the family faced and the apparent injustices to which they were subjected. Rather than improving their health, I watched, powerlessly, as it declined. This sense of ineptitude in the face of real social and economic hardships has been all too common during my early experiences in medicine.

As a medical student, I am preparing to take on the responsibilities of managing and improving the well-being of patients. Although healthcare institutions are created to improve health, it seems counterintuitive that these institutions fail to address the health-harming, oppressive forces in our society. This paradox has caused me notable moral distress during my clinical rotations as I continue to witness, first-hand, the stark health inequities experienced by many patients and communities. Rather than waiting for healthcare to establish a "standard of care" for treating social determinants of health, I have discovered, during my training, the humble power of advocacy.

Over the last year, I have had the privilege of working with an interdisciplinary team of medical providers, medical trainees, and legal professionals who, together, provide families of neonatal intensive care unit (NICU) patients with free legal services. Medical-Legal Partnerships (MLPs) are collaborations between health systems and legal organizations that aim to address the health-harming legal needs of patients. Some of these needs include unlawful evictions, employer discrimination, and habitation concerns such as black mold removal. MLPs practice preventive law to achieve health and legal justice for each patient and family. The type of impact achieved by MLPs is not only appreciable on the patient-level but also on a population-level given its upstream approach to health and its potential for legislative solutions.

I have been galvanized by the potential of policy to address individual challenges through sustainable, population-level solutions. My interest in legislation led me to other opportunities, such as taking part in the Oregon ACP (American College of Physicians) Advocacy Day Policy, Research, and Education Subcommittee. We focused on creating up-to-date educational handouts and presentations on current legislative topics, such as universal healthcare and climate change. This information was presented to attendees of the Oregon ACP Advocacy Day event and helped bolster their testimonies to the state legislature. This was a wonderful opportunity for early advocates, like myself, to begin working at the policy level.

The challenges we face as a society can be overwhelming and can produce significant moral distress, especially when one feels they lack the tools necessary for change. Moral distress is dangerous, particularly for the paralysis and resignation it can engender. However, as in my case, it can also be a necessary catalyst for action. Advocacy—whether fighting for health justice on an individual level or testifying for policy before the state legislature—is not only a productive way to find agency amid moral distress but a truly meaningful step towards a healthier and more just society.

Reflections on the Physician as Advocate

Teva Brender, MD

His handcuffs were heavier than I thought they would be. And colder too. In that moment I realized that I had never felt a real pair of handcuffs before; I certainly didn't expect the first time to be in a hospital room. After checking Mr. B's pulse, I knelt down and asked how I could help make him more comfortable. As I stepped past the correctional officer in the hallway, I paused, collecting my emotions—shock, anger, sadness—before continuing on to the nutrition room to grab him some ice water.

Biking home that night, I thought about Mr. B and the trauma he must be experiencing. As the medicine team, we could treat his sickle cell crisis and offer empathy and compassion, but benevolence alone could not palliate the indignity of being shackled to one's hospital bed.

Responsible for the full spectrum of disease and witness to the countless social determinants of health, internists are privileged with the perspective and platform to promote policies that will benefit the public. For far too long, physicians, organized medicine, and the healthcare industry have not done enough to challenge a status quo that perpetuates health disparities across race, class, wealth, and gender. Yet, times are changing. From gun violence to police brutality, structural racism, and disinformation about vaccines and COVID-19, physicians have started to find their civic voice—a legacy that I hope to inherit and continue.

But advocacy is not a solo endeavor; an effective advocate needs allies. So, days later, as I was unable to stop thinking about Mr. B, I connected with several colleagues active in the Oregon Chapter of the American College of Physicians (ACP). I had no way of knowing it at the time, but those initial conversations would eventually culminate in us writing a resolution on the healthcare rights and humane treatment of incarcerated persons that was adopted as policy by the ACP and the American Medical Association.

I am under no illusions. I first met Mr. B on my internal medicine clerkship when I was an MS3. I am currently an MS4, and just the other day I took care of a patient who was shackled to his gurney. Our resolution changed no laws, nor did it even change official policy at my institution. But, to paraphrase the great Dr. Martin Luther King Jr. who himself was drawing inspiration from 19th-century abolitionist Theodore Parker, though the moral arc of the universe bends slowly, it bends towards justice.[89] Allow me to explain.

For the last several months, I have had the privilege of co-chairing the Oregon ACP's Advocacy Day subcommittee on Policy, Research, and Education. I am now leading the same group that, just a year before, had been my introduction to policy and advocacy work. Like the old medical pedagogy—see one, do one, teach

---

89 All Things Considered. "Theodore Parker and The 'Moral Universe'". NPR. September 2010. Available at: https://www.npr.org/templates/story/story.php?storyId=129609461

one!—in this capacity, I advised a group of students who were interested in writing their own policy resolution on the reproductive healthcare rights of incarcerated females. What's more, we were able to connect them with pediatrician and State Representative Lisa Reynolds, MD, who is the chief sponsor of Oregon HB 4146, a bill to designate a gender-responsive coordinator for Oregon's correctional facilities. HB 4146 is currently being considered in the House Ways and Means Committee, so perhaps when you read this essay it will have passed and become law. If you read this essay and find that it has not passed or not made it out of committee, then understand that we still have our work cut out for us.

This is the work of the physician-advocate. Listen to our patients, both to the words that they say and the words that they don't say. Stand with our peers in order to lean on those seemingly immovable systems and structures at the root of health disparities. And bend those institutions, ever so slightly, ever so imperceptibly, towards equity and justice.

Health Equity Requires Civic Engagement: A Call to Action

Stella Safo, MD, MPH, and Eileen Barrett, MD, MPH

In a time when little feels apolitical, most would agree that every person has a right to achieve optimal health. One pathway to achieve improved health for all is by centering equity in health care delivery. The focus on health equity became more pronounced after the racial reckoning of the summer of 2020 and the resulting commitments from individuals, institutions, and companies to dismantle systemic inequities in medicine. We saw widespread support statements and an unprecedented investment in the formation of diversity, equity, and inclusion (DEI) committees. Yet despite this collective commitment, it is unclear how much has been accomplished to close the gaping inequities in healthcare outcomes that different racial and ethnic groups experience. We propose that investing in civic engagement provides one way to close the racial health gap.

What is health equity?

One challenge to implementing equitable healthcare is understanding what is meant by the term "health equity." Indeed, health equity is so widely used in current healthcare discussions that it carries many associations. We support the CDC's definition in which health equity covers the body of work needed to ensure every individual attains optimal health.[90] For those who are particularly disadvantaged because of historical and contemporary systemic inequities, implementing health equity may require additional resource allocation to that group to prioritize their needs. Health equity cannot be achieved without addressing the many social determinants of health (SDOH), which drive the worse health outcomes that minoritized racial and ethnic groups often face. These SDOH include unemployment, inadequate housing, and unsafe neighborhoods, to name a few.

How does civic engagement relate to health equity?

Addressing SDOH falls outside of the scope of work of many health systems. For instance, while we may successfully treat a patient's HIV or diabetes, we cannot guarantee access to healthful foods or safe shelter that tremendously affects health outcomes. But local municipal boards can work to address these issues. Given the reality that much of health promotion and addressing SDOH falls outside the scope of health centers and clinics, we propose that civic engagement is one mechanism that physicians and healthcare

90 CDC. "What is Health Equity." Centers for Disease Control and Prevention. 16 Dec. 2022, https://www.cdc.gov/nchhstp/healthequity/index.html

institutions must invest in to achieve health equity. We define civic engagement as encompassing the variety of ways in which individuals and groups participate in their communities and public life in service of addressing issues of public concern and/or improving community conditions.

How does civic engagement impact the health of communities?

Civic engagement is an investment in communities because it empowers those who are closest to the issues that negatively impact their health to take on the decision-making capacity that improves health outcomes. To illustrate this, let's take a look at an example in which health outcomes were directly impacted by the decisions of local elected bodies. In Flint, Michigan, public officials failed to apply corrosive inhibitors to the water supply. The result was nearly 9,000 predominantly Black children suffering from toxic levels of lead exposure. This failure of public officials to make decisions in the best interest of this population resulted in several elected leaders being tried and convicted for the water crisis that has spanned seven years. In contrast, in To'hajiilee, New Mexico, tribal and state elected officials partnered to negotiate with a private company to improve access to safe water for a rural community. These examples demonstrate what can happen to a community's health depending on how elected officials engage in health-promoting improvements. Similarly, decisions like which hospitals are closed or which neighborhoods get access to groceries with fresh fruits and vegetables all arise from advocacy and legislation that local, state, and federal elected officials oversee.

How does civic engagement help physicians?

Physicians care about patients and communities. When SDOH are addressed, patients and communities will have better health outcomes, which could be reflected in improvements in performance measures and quality scores. Additionally, many physicians are personally affected by SDOH and would directly benefit from the policy decisions that may result from a more civically engaged healthcare and patient population. Lastly, during a time when physicians have record levels of burnout, being civically engaged can help physicians exercise agency through advocacy.

How can physicians support civic engagement?

The connection between civic engagement and health has been demonstrated through various grassroots groups such as Vot-ER and Civic Health Alliance that have created a movement to provide frontline staff with resources and tools to engage patients in voter registration at the time of care. Hundreds have requested these materials to use with their patients. We've also seen physicians testify before local or federal agencies about the impact of gun violence, regressive LGBTQ policies, and reproductive rights restrictions on their patients. All of these are a form of civic engagement in healthcare.

Is civic engagement the same as being involved in politics?

In its ideal form, encouraging civic engagement is apolitical—it simply describes the process of utilizing public institutions to serve the needs of the local community. To be sure, some will see this call for physicians to become more civically engaged as a degradation of medicine's politically neutral stance. However, we believe the opposite is true. When realities like climate crises, firearms violence, or unaddressed systemic racism are negatively affecting our patients, physicians are called to act. Creating an environment within healthcare where staff and patients actively choose the elected officials who can appropriately address these issues strengthens our commitment to protect the health of our populations.

Furthermore, US law supports healthcare facilities serving as voter registration sites, therefore physicians are within the confines of their legal rights when encouraging patients and their coworkers to get registered to vote. In fact, the Internal Revenue Service and the National Voter Registration Act requires any public office that receives Medicaid dollars to offer nonpartisan voter registration booths, a little-known reality that often surprises healthcare leaders who may be reluctant to undertake voter registration for fear of legal repercussions.

Next Steps?

There is an adage that the best time to plant a tree is 30 years ago, and the next best time is today. The same holds true for physicians becoming civically engaged as a tool to improve patient health, advance health equity, improve population health, and possibly improve their own professional well-being. We may be unsure of where to begin with affecting the change we want to see. However, we should take comfort that starting with encouraging our peers, patients, and communities to invest in voting and other forms of civic engagement can drive more equitable health.

America's Gun Violence Problem Won't be Solved by Judges

Elizabeth Cerceo, MD, FACP, FHM

In a decision made by a conservative majority, the Supreme Court struck down a New York state law that restricted carrying guns in public. While the justices are throwing about esoteric debates and agonizing over semantics, I am caring for a young man today who was left quadriplegic by a gunshot wound. My colleagues have cared for victims of mass shootings. Hospital violence is rising. Mental health across the country has suffered. However, these justices prioritize giving everyone a gun to walk around with.

The institution of the courts seems to walk both sides of the fence, both encouraging widespread gun use and ownership and simultaneously, historically, enacting harsh penalties on those who use the weapons, leading the US to have more incarcerated citizens than any other country. The US contains only 5% of the global population but houses 25% of the prisoners worldwide.[91] The US

---

91 Resney, Alex. "Mass Incarceration in the United States." Ballard Brief, Jan. 2019, https:// ballardbrief.byu.edu/issue-briefs/mass-incarceration-in-the-united-states

murder rate is 25 times higher than comparable high-income countries.[92] This dichotomy begs the question of whether the justices consider these cases in a vacuum, completely divorced from the reality around them.

These conservative judges do not take care of patients. They do not personally deal with the ramifications of the theoretical decisions they pass down from a bench far removed from the American people. While physicians have been accused of not staying in our lane when it comes to gun regulation, I would like to turn the tables. There is no one better suited to weigh in on the gun debate than doctors. The scourge of gun violence is a public health crisis.

On the other hand, judges who consider a ruling in the absence of its implications are acting without regard to the health and well-being of the Americans this institution was created to protect. The judges consider the right to live a life without being gunned down as a lesser good than being able to carry a gun in public. This reasoning seems fatally flawed.

Their reasoning is, by their own admission, predicated on a historical interpretation of the Second Amendment, but the problem today is gun violence—not colonial invaders. We are not talking about bayonets and crossbows but, rather, concealed handguns in busy shopping malls and in subway stations. The conservative justices refuse to acknowledge the ills of our current society and have weakened the institution they represent.

That the American people are subject to the whims of these unelected officials is unconscionable. While this branch of government is meant to be part of a system of checks and balances, SCOTUS

---

92 Grinshteyn, Erin and David Hemenway. "Violent Death Rates: The US Compared with Other High-income OECD Countries." *The American Journal of Medicine*, vol. 129, no. 3, Mar 2016, pp. 266-73. doi: 10.1016/j.amjmed.2015.10.025.

has been embracing without hindrance ever more far-reaching legislation with potentially severely negative consequences. Where are the checks and balances for decisions which may go against the public good or at the very least public opinion? We did not vote for these justices who are in place. We had no say in the individuals who now hold sway over the outcomes for many and who will be ensconced on that bench for years to come. Even many conservatives in favor of gun protections question the wisdom of promoting a gun on every hip in every restaurant, library, grocery store, and hospital.

Certainly, the Senate passage of a bipartisan gun safety bill may act to counter some of the harm incurred. Perhaps states such as New Jersey will scramble to come up with legislation to work around the Supreme Court decision. While they do, America's gun violence problem will continue to worsen. Doctors, nurses, and other health professionals will deal with the consequences firsthand while the Supreme Court debates historical context. America's gun violence problem won't be solved by judges; the solution—and action—starts with us.

Gun Violence is Being Normalized: A Call for Gun Reform

Montserrat Tijerina, BA

As a first-year medical student observing in a Chicago pediatric ICU, I couldn't help noticing the constant stream of people going in and out of one of the patient rooms. After minutes of wondering, I walked over to my nurse and asked about the child.

"Gunshot wound to the head. She's brain-dead. They will be pulling the plug in the next few hours."

I shoved my emotions aside before I could feel anything. We had to see our next patient. So I numbed myself even as I heard the cries of the little child's family echo down the hall.

"Compartmentalize," I told myself. "Don't think too much about it."

But today, I imagine the 19 children shot in Uvalde, Texas, and I can no longer force back my feelings. I have no numbness left to give. The leading cause of death for children between the ages of 1-19 years old is firearm-related death.[93] Each day in the United

93 Goldstick, Jason E. et al. "Current Causes of Death in Children and Adolescents in the United States." *New England Journal of Medicine,* vol. 386, no. 20, May 2022, pp. 1955-1956. doi: 10.1056/NEJMc2201761

States, about 19 children die or are treated in the ED for a firearm injury.[94] It's time we treat gun violence as a preventable public health issue.

Let's rewind a bit.

It's August 2019. A gunman targets Latino communities in El Paso, Texas. He kills 23 people and injures 25 others at a Walmart. A week after the El Paso shooting, another gunman kills 7 people and injures 25 others in Midland-Odessa. Texas mourns. Texas demands action.

Governor Abbott promised. "Never again," he said.

In response, he and the Texas legislature implemented eight executive orders, SB 11, and HB 1387 in September of 2019. The executive orders address the mass shootings in El Paso and Midland-Odessa and focus on improving reporting channels amongst law enforcement and the public when someone is deemed a threat or a concern for violence.

On the other hand, SB 11 and HB 1387 are primarily a response to the 2018 fatal shooting at Santa Fe High School that killed 13 students. SB 11 aims to increase mental health support in schools, requires easy classroom access to telephones, and establishes threat assessment teams that work to identify students who may pose a danger to school safety. HB 1387 removes the limit on the number of trained teachers and staff who can carry guns on public school grounds.

What's baffling is the immediate response to mitigate—*not eradicate*—the threat of gun violence. Why improve reporting channels when stricter background checks can be put in place? Why create threat assessment teams that have the potential to

94 Fowler, Katherine A et al. "Childhood Firearm Injuries in the United States." *Pediatrics*, vol. 140, no. 1, 2017, e20163486. doi: 10.1542/peds.2016-3486

profile students based on their race, ethnicity, and disabled status when we could work to ensure that guns, especially AR-15's, do not reach the hands of teens not even old enough to grab a glass of beer? And it shouldn't be lost on us that the high school teen who killed the children at Robb Elementary had purchased two rifles days after his 18th birthday, had recently made threats against his own classmates, and had been cutting scars on his face—all during Mental Health Awareness Month. Where are the mental health resources that Governor Abbott vowed to support?

"We know that words alone are inadequate," Abbott said in response to many of these massacres. "Words must be met with action."

And action, he took. In September of 2021, HB 1927 went into effect in Texas. It allows people who legally qualify and who are over 21 years old to publicly carry a gun without a license to carry. That same month, Texas named itself a "Second Amendment sanctuary state" as a means of banning state and local governments from implementing specific gun legislation coming from the federal level. The Texas legislature also passed SB 19 and HB 1500, which prohibits state and local contracts that "discriminate against the firearm and ammunition industries" and terminates the governor's power to restrict gun sales during emergencies, respectively.

Fast-forward to May 24, 2022. It's a normal morning at Robb Elementary School. Students pass the school sign. "Welcome, Bienvenidos." Summer break is just two days away. Parents cheer for their children as they watch the students' honor roll ceremony. Many of these kids would be heading to Flores Middle School in August. Time flies: the children are growing up. *Qué orgullo.*

These are the last moments many parents spent with their children—hugging them, telling them how proud they are of them.

Just a few more hours changed everything, forever, because of 18-year-old Salvador Ramos. Ramos shot 19 children and 2 teachers, who will never see their families again. These kids will never go to Flores Middle School. They will never attend a high school graduation. They will never live the lives we should have done better to protect. Their families will never be the same.

My questions for the Texas legislature: How do your state laws help our communities? Who or what are you really protecting?

The reality is that the state and federal governments must do more. Ten people in Buffalo were targeted and killed. A church in California was gunned. At least 22 people in Texas were massacred.

But hey—it's just another two weeks in the United States.

Legislators tweet words. They mourn for a few days, and they send their thoughts and prayers to the families who want so much more from them. They go back to work, and they make firearms readily accessible for anyone to carry anywhere.

Wake up. Our children are dying. And somehow, we numb ourselves to it—again, and again.

As I prepare to become a doctor at the Pritzker School of Medicine, I refuse to become desensitized to the innocent deaths of children, mothers, fathers, and community members. I refuse to shove my emotions to the side and bottle up my agony in the face of such senseless violence. I refuse to normalize mass shootings.

Gun reform must start **now**. Take a moment to feel your full range of emotions, then call or write to your local legislators.

Women Physicians on Mother Earth

Elizabeth Cerceo, MD, FACP, FHM

If you're going to be a feminist on a hot planet,
you have to be a climate feminist.

—KATHARINE K. WILKINSON, CO-EDITOR

OF THE CLIMATE ANTHOLOGY *ALL WE CAN SAVE*[95]

I've always considered myself an environmentalist, but I did not get truly passionate/slightly obsessed until I had children. I cannot exactly explain why I wasn't more fired up before that, because I certainly cared. As a child, I remember my father, a chemist, used to have jars around the yard to collect rainwater. My brother and I used to make fun of the precious collection, but he was measuring levels of acid rain. He made us turn off the lights religiously, and the house was always a little too hot in the summer because the thermostat was off limits. I still had these habits deeply embedded in my psyche, but I didn't picture myself marching in protests. We cannot dwell on the past but only move forward.

---

95 Johnson, Ayana Elizabeth and Katharine K. Wilkinson. *All We Can Save: Truth, Courage, & Solutions for the Climate Crisis.* One World, 2021.

Whether we think of ourselves as privileged or not, many physicians or physician families fall into the "1%" category of over $450,000 or close to it. We have a personal responsibility with our actions, such as not switching out our gas-guzzler SUVs every couple of years, not throwing away our clothes, and cutting down on air travel. Even if we all lived like monks, though, policy change is what will restructure our world. We need to be active. We, as physicians, have an incredibly powerful voice that we can raise in defense of this planet and the people on it.

Women have a unique role in this. Much of the force behind these climate movements have come from behind. They have been started by people without a voice, like teenagers who cannot vote—usually girls, many of whom are LGBTQ—and they have changed the conversation. I do not mean to say that men are not passionate about the future of our planet as well but look at the COP26 talks in Glasgow. Many of the world leaders at the table are old and male whereas the protests are led largely by young women. Women have not traditionally been at the table to challenge the status quo. The same is true for people of color, Indigenous people, and young people.

These young women speak with a passion and fury that comes with the realization of the attendant suffering that comes with dragging our feet. In fact, emissions of greenhouse gases have risen more since the first international climate summit 27 years ago than all of human history. Now, scientists say the world has less than a decade to sharply curtail emissions to avert the worst climate consequences.

Young women from around the world recognize that women are more impacted by the climate crisis than men, especially low-income women with children to feed. When there are climate disasters, women are also more impacted. There is an increase in violence against women when husbands are stressed from crop failures or drought. Women are subjected to assaults when they must travel long distances to get water and food. Refugee camps are notoriously unsafe for women and girls. Early marriages and sex trafficking can all result. Education of women and girls in developing nations is a shared goal with the climate movement, as girls cannot go to school when they must help their poor families.

If we think the Global North is to be spared, we are wrong. The Pentagon has called climate a "threat multiplier" in that it exacerbates already existing disparities and injustices. Besides its impact on the social determinants of health, air pollution contributes to 350,000 premature deaths in the US alone[96] and over 10 million globally. These are our patients, not to mention our neighbors, our parents, and our children. It has been associated with everything from cardiopulmonary disease to cognitive decline, from adverse birth outcomes to criminality. It impacts nearly every condition we seek to treat.

So, what can we do?

Pick one thing, do it once a week, and things will change. Green your hospital or ambulatory practice. Work with your medical societies to advocate for environmental justice. The American College of Physicians and the American Lung Association are just two of the active societies. The American Society of Anesthesiologists started an Inhaled Anesthetic 2020 Challenge as part of an internation-

---

96 Vohra, Karn et al. "Global mortality from outdoor fine particle pollution generated by fossil fuel combustion: Results from GEOS-Chem." *Environmental Research*, vol. 195, Apr 2021, pp. 110754. doi: 10.1016/j.envres.2021.110754.

al campaign to decrease these potent greenhouse gasses.[97] Write op-eds. Teach the impacts of health and climate change to your medical students, to your colleagues, your patients, and anyone who will listen. Advocate for climate change education in your children's schools.

You can also join nonphysician campaigns or activist groups like Citizens' Climate Lobby, the Sunrise Movement, 350.org, or maybe Extinction Rebellion. You can join the Sierra Club, League of Conservation Voters, or League of Women Voters. Donate money. Sunrise Movement, Fridays for Future (Greta Thunberg's organization), and Greenpeace are some worthy organizations. Groups with an environmental justice focus include the Centre for Social Justice, Uprose, and We Act. Climate Power and Evergreen Action are writing climate policy. The Environmental Voter Project and Stacey Abrams' Fair Fight Action focus on voting rights to affect climate change policy. Greenfaith is a faith-based environmental organization. Talk about climate change in your social networks, even when it seems uncomfortable. And, of course, a simple thing is to vote in every election, national and local! Once they are in office, call their offices, email them, and thank them for their support.

As women in medicine, we cannot just amplify messages. We can lead the way and support women's empowerment as a strategy to improve the environmental resilience of our communities.

Don't be quiet; be persistent. There is too much at stake.

---

97 Sherman, Jodi D. et al. "Inhaled Anesthetic 2020 Challenge: Reduce Your Inhaled Anesthetic Carbon Emissions by 50%!" *ASA Monitor* 2020, vol. 84, Apr. 2020, pp. 14–17.

Chapter 10
COVID-19

Remember When

Angela Roberts Selzer, MD

Remember when they cheered for us?
When they clapped their hands for us?
Flew over, drove by, and cheered for us?
We were terrified and tired, but they appreciated us.
Now they jeer at us.
Refuse a free vaccine to endanger us.
Argue and protest and sneer at us.
Then get sick and, in fear, come back to us.
Gasping for air as they plead with us.
We ignore the hate to be with them.
Always provide the best care for them.
Though a vaccine alone could have kept them at home.
We fight for their lives and again risk our own.
How much longer can we do this?
It's not clear to us.
They don't care for us.
Remember when they cheered for us?

What Happened to Public Health?

Shoshana N. Benjamin, MPH

I was in my second semester of my master's of public health in New York City when the COVID-19 pandemic started. And aside from all of the fear and anxiety I was experiencing because of the pandemic, I remember feeling so proud that I had chosen the field of public health. While many of us would agree that the early response to COVID-19, especially with 20-20 hindsight (no pun intended) was severely lacking, I was excited that the major tenets of public health—prevention and promotion—were taking center stage.

For my summer practicum that year, I worked for the New York City Department of Health and Mental Hygiene, helping to craft messaging about COVID-19 and equity. It was inspiring to be a part of an organization dedicated to protecting my city. During a Zoom happy hour with friends, I darkly joked that the one upside of the pandemic was that at least people now knew what public health was.

But things have changed—especially still as I write this in Fall 2022.

Since the first waves of the pandemic, we've seen a terrifying about-face from health professionals—or health professionals who do not have appropriate training portraying themselves as experts in public health. You know that we are in crisis when medical doctors who are ostensibly public health-focused are calling for a return to "normal" as they minimize the risk of COVID. The Centers for Disease Control and Prevention (CDC) is barely calling for any COVID-19 *population*-level mitigation measures, focusing only on reducing severe disease through vaccination and treatment (though barely doing any messaging about the updated, bivalent boosters) and especially focusing on *individual* risk assessment and reduction. The CDC has forgotten its name and its mandate: to control and prevent disease.

During orientation for grad school, a professor told us the classic public health parable about people in the river. Basically, someone sees that there are people drowning in a river and immediately starts scooping them out. Another person runs upstream to see why there are all these people in the river, only to find a broken bridge. Obviously, it's critical to get the people out of the river, but it's more efficient (and less traumatizing for the people) to fix the bridge and keep them from getting into the river in the first place. That's what public health is about: preventing people from getting into the river; preventing people from getting sick in the first place.

We had the tools to prevent people from getting COVID in the first place: increasing indoor ventilation, masking (with high-quality masks) indoors, mandating boosters, making testing free and easily available, etc. And we need to use everything in our arsenal to prevent COVID infection in the first place, not just severe disease as a complication. Long COVID is a clear and present risk that we know about; data suggests that between 20-30% of people who are infected with COVID develop long COVID. And that is what we know. What we don't know is what will happen to people who've gotten COVID in a year, five years, a decade, or longer. It can take HIV years to turn into AIDS, chicken pox can flare as shingles after decades, and EBV can lead to multiple sclerosis. In addition to the mass disabling that is occurring due to Long COVID, what potential horror awaits us down the road? HPV turns into multiple types of cancer (cervical, head/neck, and anal): Will COVID lead to nothing or another terrible disease? Already, evidence demonstrates that COVID is a vascular disease and can lead to cardiac and neurologic complications. The truth is we don't know, and because of that we must be careful. We must prevent every infection we can.

When I go on Twitter and see medical professionals down-playing the risk of COVID and advocating against masks or other protective measures, or when the CDC opts to let millions of Americans die or become disabled, I feel betrayed. As someone who is still taking COVID fairly seriously, I always wear a KN95 or N95 when inside public spaces, I don't eat indoors at restaurants, and I only hang out unmasked inside with friends if we've all taken rapids or gotten PCRs. I feel gaslit by the government and medical pundits. The pandemic is still happening, with hundreds of Americans dying every day, but sometimes it feels like there is an ever-shrinking minority who both acknowledges that or thinks we should do something about it.

We need to return to public health, to thinking about how to protect populations instead of relying on people's individual choices. We need to go upstream and keep people from ending up in the river in the first place.

You Broke Us

Kate Ropp, MD

We wanted to help people
We were smart and driven
We loved science and physiology, humans and disease
So, we made a commitment
We signed up
It was an honor
We read thousands of pages
Attended hundreds of lectures
Pulled all-nighters
Took more exams than we thought possible
Finals week felt insurmountable
But it didn't break us
It made us stronger
We learned statistics and biochemistry
Immunology and pathophysiology
We mastered genetics, virology and pharmacology
We read scientific papers and learned how to dissect them
Papers, not videos

It was an honor
We came running when you needed us
Literally, running down the hallway
To the ICU, the trauma bay, labor and delivery
I need help, you said
We can help, we said
It was an honor
There were moments that we thought would break us
Moments that drove us to journaling, to therapy, to nightmares
Broken babies.
Paralyzed children.
Dead pregnant mothers with three kids at home.
The wail of a mother whose son just died.
We bent but we did not break
We returned because you needed us
And we could help
It was an honor
Then there was fear
Fear of walking into our place of work
Fear that we'd be killed by going to work
Fear that we'd kill a loved one because of our work
There were tears and sleepless nights and anti-anxiety medications
But you banged your pots and pans
You sent us pizzas and called us heroes
You needed us
We could help
So we wore our masks, and our gowns, and our gloves, and our goggles

We decontaminated ourselves before going home and isolated ourselves from our families

We almost broke

It was an honor

How quickly the joy of vaccine victory turned to defeat

Elation to rage

You've learned to do your own research now

You know better than we do

Gaslighting is your language

Your selfishness is astounding

You don't want our help when we ask you to stay healthy

Yet, you arrive at our doors begging for help at the end

You stole our resources

You hobbled our ability to help those who did what they were supposed to do

You killed our patients by filling our beds and using up our ventilators

We can't help any more

You broke us

There is no more honor

Reflections on the COVID-19 Pandemic*

Amy Comander, MD, DipABLM

One night in early 2022, my husband and I did something we had not done in quite some time: we went out for dinner at our favorite sushi restaurant in Brookline, Massachusetts.

We had not been there since early 2020! It felt great to have a night out alone (our children were occupied), enjoy our dinner, and reclaim a sense of normalcy.

Unfortunately, it was only a sense of normalcy as we were then two years into the pandemic. The first case of COVID-19 in the US was reported on January 21, 2020. Does it feel longer or shorter? Either way, our lives have been fundamentally changed.

As of March 6, 2022, there have been 6 million deaths around the world and nearly 1 million deaths in the U.S. In the US, this represents the death of about 0.3% of the entire population, or one in 340 people. In the US, there are just more than 600,000 deaths from cancer each year.

Although COVID-19 cases from the Omicron wave are thankfully sharply down in Massachusetts, daily deaths then still exceed

1,000 people per day nationally. The loss of lives during this time is incomprehensible.

Still, it does feel as if our world is opening again. But what happens next? How do we return to normalcy? What will be our next chapter?

An Unsettling Time

Although the loss of life is devastating to comprehend, the pandemic has fundamentally changed us in many ways.

I am a breast oncologist at Massachusetts General Cancer Center. Working as a physician during the COVID-19 pandemic has been the most difficult challenge of my career. I know many colleagues have similar sentiments with many of us temporarily being reassigned to treat inpatients with COVID-19.

During this unsettling time, we have had to learn how to care for patients with COVID-19 while also ensuring the safety of patients with cancer at our hospital. Although oncology treatment is challenging enough, it has been even more challenging to help our patients navigate new, uncharted waters.

How much does the risk/benefit ratio of neutropenia change during each phase of a respiratory pandemic? Besides the obvious fears of infection and dangers of infection, we faced other unforeseen obstacles. When would my patient, newly diagnosed with operable breast cancer, get to have her surgery? How can a cancer operation be considered elective? What is an appropriate treatment protocol in the setting of a pandemic? To what lengths should patients go to protect themselves when they have compromised immune systems?

To make our clinics as safe as possible, the care for our patients with cancer was fundamentally changed for many months.

Our patients could not have a family member or friend join them at appointments. Many times, I found myself seeing a patient, newly diagnosed with breast cancer, all by herself, with a partner or friend present via FaceTime on a smartphone.

Our patients in the hospital could not have visitors because this could place them, and other patients, at risk for exposure to COVID-19. Our inpatients were alone all day in the hospital. This was unsettling, especially for those who were very ill.

And yet I recall attending one of the weekly Massachusetts General Hospital (MGH) Schwartz Rounds, sponsored by the Schwartz Center for Compassionate Healthcare. I will never forget the words of one of my nursing colleagues who commented that "hospitalized patients are not alone since they have us."

Staying Grounded Amid Uncertainty

As we continue to navigate the twists and turns of the pandemic, I know each of us will continue to reflect on the experiences of these past years and ponder the next chapter ahead.

In early 2022, our Women in Oncology group at MGH invited Nancy Rappaport, MD, child psychiatrist and associate professor of psychiatry at Harvard Medical School, to speak about "What Cancer and a Pandemic Can Teach Us about Navigating Uncertainty." One of her important messages that resonated with me is the recognition that we have learned to "stay grounded in the present moment while dancing with uncertainty."

Learning how to "navigate uncertainty" is certainly a challenge that our patients face after receiving a diagnosis of cancer, and I have learned many lessons of strength and resilience from my own patients over the years. I am hopeful that the lessons I have learned from my own patients, and from this difficult time, will help me navigate further challenges ahead.

I recall another comment during that MGH Schwartz Rounds from the spring of 2020. A nursing colleague commented, "The only thing more formidable than these scary past few weeks is the incessant outpouring of kindness, compassion, and teamwork that have been displayed throughout this time of crisis. Love will always conquer fear. Better days are coming, and we will get through this together."

* *This piece comes from the partnership between the WIMS Blog and the Healio Women in Oncology blog:*

Comander A. Women in Oncology (blog): Reflections on the COVID-19 pandemic. Healio, March 8, 2022. Available at: https://www.wimedicine.org/blog/reflections-on-the-covid-19-pandemic. Reprinted with permission from Healio.

Changing the Culture of Immunization

Nadine Gartner, JD

For far too long, the general public has associated immunizations with fear: fear of needles, fear of the unknown (e.g., ingredients or how vaccines work), and fear of side-effects. Most medical professionals, on the other hand, view immunizations as one of the safest and most effective interventions available to us. So, how can we bridge the gap between public perception and the medical world's understanding? The answer is to change the culture of immunization from fear to love. Here, I share my position as a nonclinician, empowered woman, and head of a vaccine advocacy organization.

No More Needles

Changing the culture of immunization begins with the words and images we employ. First and foremost: *stop using images of needles.* No one likes needles. No one sees a needle and thinks, "Yes! Please stab me now!" An analysis by researchers at the University of Michigan showed that 20-30% of adults cited concern about needles.[98] There is no need to use images of needles on flyers, social media, or any other outreach you're doing to promote immunizations. Use pictures of band-aids, vaccine vials, hearts, or a myriad of other things instead. And, if you see local media using graphics of needles, tell them why it's hurting our attempts at building healthier communities.

Lead with Love and Empathy

Second, lead with love and empathy when discussing immunizations. If you're a clinician, use motivational interviewing techniques to pinpoint the patient's concern. Doing so ensures that your patient feels heard and confirms what you need to address. Imagine yourself as a journalist or anthropologist and ask a lot of questions: What are your concerns? Where did you hear that? Who do you trust for medical information? You want to meet people where they are and, together, guide them toward evidence-based resources.

Transform with Positivity

Third, transform your environment into a confident immunization space. Post images and videos of happy people doing things they love with positive messages about immunizations throughout your clinic, children's schools, and on social media. Place buttons on your lapels or bags that proudly share your immunization status. Ask your children's schools about their vaccination rates and encourage them to adopt sensible immunization policies. Become a peer advocate and learn how to educate your specific community

---

98 McLenon, Jennifer and Mary AM Rogers. "The fear of needles: A systematic review and meta-analysis." *Journal of Advanced Nursing*, vol. 75, no. 1, Jan. 2019, pp. 30-42. doi: 10.1111/jan.13818

about vaccines. Be open with your friends and family about your and your children's vaccination status and ask about their own. Let's normalize sharing this information, just as we do with food allergies, so that we can best protect our children and communities.

How to Handle the Anti-Vaccine Crowd

What if your patient or loved one falls into the truly anti-vaccine crowd and is not merely vaccine-hesitant? Be an approachable and nonjudgmental presence for the person by asking questions and responding with kindness. Don't debate or ridicule the falsehoods. Ask questions that poke holes and prompt the person to reconsider their assumptions. Above all else, be patient and reach out frequently so that the person feels cared for and tethered to a real-life relationship as opposed to an online conspiracy network.

Spread the Truth

Vaccines only work when the entire community participates. Use "community immunity" rather than "herd immunity," which turns people off because of the animal connotation. It's on all of us to ensure that immunizations are available, accessible, and desirable. Changing the public's perception is critical to achieve that goal. Let love be your guide as you proudly spread the truth about immunizations.

Camp Edition, Summer 2021

Avital O'Glasser, MD, FACP, SFHM, DFPM

Yes, I sent my kid to sleepaway camp in the summer of 2021.

Three weeks away from home during the second summer of a global pandemic, three glorious, special, amazing weeks of being a kid, surrounded by other kids and reclaiming what he had missed the prior summer.

My oldest needed to go to sleep away camp. He just had to! I'm not saying this because he needed time away from our intense, bubbled, family experience, or needed a long break from screen time, or because his younger brother needed a chance to be an only child for three weeks. Well, those are all true but they weren't the driving reasons. My husband and I stand by every decision we have made to keep our kids safe during this pandemic and we knew, and *trusted*, that sending him to camp was the right decision.*

Planning for summer 2021, and the anticipation of being able to attend, began almost as soon as we received word of cancellations in spring 2020. Canceling camp was a difficult decision and the right one to make.

For full transparency, I joined the camp's Board of Directors last fall and then became the chair of its medical committee. Some days I wondered why I took on this role with my limited spare time as a physician-mom living and working during a pandemic. However, this camp is an incredibly special part of my family and our community. Giving my time to support the camp, to reinforce its core values of community engagement and collective responsibility, and to role model sound responses to the pandemic was the right way to spend my time.

Planning for a successful summer 2021 began early in 2020. It took energy, effort, resources, advocacy, activism, leadership, communication, community engagements, creativity, and trust—skills necessary to any element of pandemic response. It included the innovative leadership of the camp's executive director to form the Washington State Camp Coalition to bring camp leadership together and to work closely with the governor's office and public health officials. It took intimate knowledge of the guidance provided by the American Camp Association.

We convened the robust, interdisciplinary medical committee early in 2021, even before many healthcare professionals had received their second COVID vaccine dose. As the months counted down to drop-off day, we had more reasons to be cautiously optimistic—vaccine eligibility for educators and camp staff, widespread vaccinations for adults, vaccines for 16 and older, and finally vaccines for 12 and older about a month before camp started.

Even as reports began to trickle in of summer camp outbreaks elsewhere in the country, we retained our sense of trust—trust in our planning, trust in the science and the protocols, trust in the guidance from the state and professional organizations, trust in the camp leadership and its staff, and trust in our community to do their part before sending their kids. Entry to camp required negative test results and low-risk behavior in the days preceding arrival. Once on site, everyone went through screening testing multiple times. Staff had to be vaccinated and had new limitations for day-off activities. Podding, social distancing between individual bunks, masking, daily symptom screening, and low thresholds for symptom-based testing were all implemented. The mental health support was also ramped up, anticipating that "re-entry" might be challenging for some kids.

The first round of universal screening tests came back once, then twice for session one. We repeated that success for session two, and then session three.

My kiddo, who attended session one, came home over a month ago—tired, dirty, and incredibly happy. By the time I wrote this essay, camp had officially ended for the summer.

They did it. Camp did it. We did it. Our community did it.

A COVID-free summer of 2021 was not easy but it was doable through the combination of leadership, proactive planning, organization, community engagement, and trust. Had we been facing the Delta variant surge at the beginning of the summer, would we have been as successful? I honestly don't know. But I do know that hundreds of kids got to be kids with each other for weeks this summer. And I know that my kiddo will be going back next summer.

In fact, our early bird registration is already complete.

* I am not revealing the name of the camp to protect my children's privacy.

Summer 2022–My COVID Travelog

Naomi Leavitt

In July 2022, I was getting our family ready to leave on a trip that we had been planning for almost three years: three weeks in the Netherlands, where I was born, to see family and to meet four new babies who had been born to cousins since our last visit.

My husband and I had spent so much time, energy, and brain cells on our daily choices since March 2020. Is the party outside? Are the people vaccinated? Will guests be masked at the community event? Will there be a Zoom option? We didn't hug our parents for thirteen months. We didn't have any guests over for holiday meals or celebrations. We said no to countless events and invitations because it meant less of a risk of getting COVID. We kept to our unit of four, and our world became very small. We did our very best to keep everyone safe with smart choices.

Since the beginning of COVID, we have masked in public indoor settings and often did in busy outdoor settings too. We packed so many masks and rapid COVID tests for our trip. The week leading up to our departure we were extra careful with events and parties.

We had decided we would mask at the airports, on the planes, on public transportation, and in museums and stores. We were so elated and grateful to have the chance to finally travel to the Netherlands again.

Our adjustment to the nine-hour time zone difference was rough. I am used to being a cranky zombie for the first two days: I power through and always turn out fine. But the persistence of jet lag four days into the trip prompted a rapid COVID test. Within two minutes, it was clearly positive. Here I was, in the middle of Amsterdam, after two and a half years of being so incredibly cautious, and I had COVID. The virus doesn't know where I am or how much the Airbnb cost.

I said a lot of bad words and immediately switched gears. I moved all of my things plus a bunch of water bottles into one of the bedrooms, which became my world. I had my meals in my room or outside. I had my own bathroom. We were able to juggle the rooms enough so that I could stay separate and keep my family safe. I *never* expected the masks that we packed would be worn inside of our house to protect my husband and kids from me!

I had a lot of time to think and simply be. I tried to welcome and allow any and all emotions. They were all completely legitimate. How did this happen? Where could I have gotten it? Most likely the plane or the airport. I had spent ten hours with hundreds of other people on the same plane.

I was an angry person and stymied mom. I was in one of my favorite cities in the world and I couldn't leave the house or hug my kids good night. I felt stuck and furious. I had planned and been flexible and thought through all of the details. Now, I was simply trying to drink a ton of water and stay away from my family by keeping to my bedroom.

I was truly indebted to the friends who generously offered their professional medical knowledge when I was scrambling and feeling very alone. I had Dutch family and friends reach out with phone numbers, clinic names, websites, and just plain, old moral support. One family even sent flowers and chocolate to our door. The folks back home were sending memes, jokes, and videos galore to keep me sane.

We tried to salvage our trip while being truly focused on the safety of our kids, who continued to test negative. On day eleven, I tested negative. My youngest daughter jumped onto me for the biggest snuggle ever once she heard the news.

Our trip resumed, possibly at a slower pace, and certainly with a different focus. The museums weren't going anywhere. It was about our family and friends at this point—our trip became people focused. We savored every little moment, every car ride, every interaction with the neighbors and their dogs, every sunset, every gelato. In the end, we managed to see every single family member in the Netherlands. Even with ten days lost to COVID chaos, we packed in a tremendous time in the land of cheese and bicycles.

And our kids remained COVID-negative. That masking and staying away and taking isolation and quarantine seriously worked. All of the scrambling and room flipping and buying of new toothbrushes was worth it. I was stunned and grateful and humbled.

My vacation time also gave me a chance to rest and think and process the whirlwind. I am a planner and a thinker and an overthinker, and yet there was still so much that I didn't consider or plan for. As so many of us dip our toes back into travel or jump into what we have been doing for a while, I hope we can keep sight of some basic things.

1. Pack masks and tests, even if you don't mask, even if you're in a place with a CVS and Walgreens on every street corner. You don't want to have to bumble to a store if someone isn't feeling well, and you don't want to find out every place is out of stock. Yep, it will take up some space in your luggage, but it may save your sanity in the possibility that they are needed.

2. Know the protocols and standards of the place you are going to. Be familiar with the government websites that show all of this and if possible, have a local contact or two as a resource, especially if you don't speak the native language.

3. Have backup plans and then more plans. Know where people would sleep, eat, which bathrooms would be for those who are sick, and have a second lodging place or hotel as a "sick house" if needed. Have some of these written down or shared on Google Docs so in case you, the planner, are the one who is sick, someone else can take over. If you have really young kids, think of who would care for them if both you and your partner end up sick. Know where and how groceries and other supplies would get to you if you're in isolation.

The world has changed so much and keeps changing. I am so incredibly grateful for the trip we had, despite a crazy, huge challenge at the beginning. I hope we can all continue to make progress carefully and wisely. I wish for each of us to be honest and to share and to be real about our struggles and our accomplishments. Here's to more of us living safely.

Making Memories, Saving Memories

Avital O'Glasser, MD, FACP, SFHM, DFPM

I flipped through our photo albums that displayed a stark difference between pre-pandemic life and pandemic life. I was twenty months behind in updating the albums. I love photo albums because I grew up in a family of photographers. I've maintained the habit of keeping photo albums myself. I realized that the last photo album I made included pictures through December 2019, which means the last eighteen months of photos I needed to catch up on were from the COVID-19 Pandemic. I wasn't sure if I wanted to put pandemic photos in my cherished albums, but it was time. It was part of life. But it wasn't easy to add them.

That stark contrast between our pre-pandemic life and our pandemic life was unsettling—the last couple's trip my husband and I took in January 2020, the last time my kids were on a plane in February 2020, the last selfie with friends at the 2020 ACGME conference (on February 28, 2020—the day the first case of COVID was diagnosed in Oregon), the last dinner-and-theater date night we had on March 7, 2020.

In March 2020, when we thought lockdown would be an intense few weeks, I took pictures of everything. Everything! I felt so compelled to save it in the moment—almost as if I couldn't believe what was happening in real time, because so much of it was both unbelievable and a blur.

I photographed every change we made to the house to support two homeschooling kids, and every creative dish we concocted out of what we had in the pantry and chest freezer when grocery delivery services were booking out a week. I screen-grabbed GIFs, memes, text message conversations, and emails with critical updates.

I had plenty of excuses to be twenty months behind on catching up on photo albums. I was busy, I was stressed, I could barely keep my eyes open most nights after we put the kids to bed. I also realized it was going to be tough and emotional. Even flipping through the photos on my phone was often tough. Then I realized that just because something is tough doesn't mean we shouldn't remember it. Indeed, a wise person once said those who forget the past are doomed to repeat it. It was critically important to preserve the early (and middle . . . and ongoing . . .) pandemic memories as much as possible. I needed to preserve these family members.

So, I sat down and caught up on photo albums. Into them the memories went. The basement cleanup to make learning space for homeschool. The bookshelf with all the various puzzle and logic books for "learning time" because we didn't know what virtual instruction school would pull together. A screen grab of the email from work declaring mandatory telecommuting. A screen grab of an email from my husband's woodworking guild calling for N95 donations. Signs at our neighborhood small businesses as they pivoted to online shopping and curbside pickup. A collage of the numerous thousand-piece puzzles we completed. My kids wearing handsewn masks for the first time. A picture of the first sardine dish we crafted in late March because we raided the emergency food kit—along with a picture of the internet search for "do sardines ever go bad," as they had expired two months prior.

My kids have entered the "stop taking my picture, Mommy!" phase, but I think to myself, "You'll want to see this in ten years, in five years, in one year! You're going to want to remember what you did, what we did as a family, to get through this pandemic together, to build our resilience, to discover and nurture new hobbies, and to stay safe." They squealed with delight looking through the photo albums when they arrived. I encourage you to do the same.

That sardine dish has become a family staple. Its creation is cemented in family history and, for the record, we did not get food poisoning that night.

Chapter 11
THE "ANTI"S

George Floyd Found Allies in His Community and in Physicians

Marie Ayorkor Laryea, MD, MDCM, FRCPC

Mr. Rogers famously spoke of his mother telling him to look for the helpers when something on the news scared him; however, the helpers were on George Floyd on the day he died.

I have only watched the video of George Floyd's death once. That call to a departed mother. *Mama.* With that one word, it seemed I had witnessed the murder of a child, and it was unbearable to watch. I was overwhelmed with a feeling I had only ever felt once before.

In medical school, a patient I was admitting suffered papillary muscle rupture and died in front of me. When they took their last breath, I felt panic. I felt I should be acting. I turned on the oxygen and rushed to press the mask to the patient's face well after that oxygen could do any good. The feeling that inaction is intolerable is the exact feeling I had watching that horrific video. It was like the ABCs in reverse. First, they compromise the airway. Then, the breathing ceases. Then, the man is pulseless.

I also found the trial very difficult to watch but for very different reasons. The trial showed the actors killing George Floyd as depraved, callous, and immoral. Unexpected, however, were other thoughts I had watching witnesses testify for the prosecution.

The witnesses all appeared traumatized and I understood well when they spoke of inaction feeling wrong. Those everyday people who filmed, or tried to intervene, were not able to save him that day. However, they helped the prosecutors piece together a case, helped the Floyd family get some measure of justice, and helped the nation restore its faith in community and humanity. They helped show our children what compassion looks like, what civic duty means, and what caring for others takes. Seeing all those engaged people trying to help Mr. Floyd likely offered some solace to his family, too. He did not die alone in the custody of a man who thought of him as subhuman. He was also surrounded by his concerned community trying to help him.

In that courtroom, something very meaningful for our profession also happened. Physicians were there, on the witness stand, playing their part in obtaining justice for the man none of us were allowed to help. Physicians reviewed facts, explained findings, and educated the court in nontechnical language about restrictive respiratory defects, oxygenation, atherosclerosis, left ventricular hypertrophy, incidentalomas, and pharmacology. Pulmonology and Critical Care. Cardiology. Pathology. Toxicology. Emergency Medicine. Doctors came forward and did what we all do in clinic every day: explain complex disease in simple terms and educate. They were all part of George Floyd's justice team and they made me singularly proud to be a peer.

Although institutions often fall short and racism in health care is a real thing many of us face daily, the case of George Floyd reminded me of the power of medicine even when we are powerless to heal. We can witness. We can advocate. We can support. We are part of that community witnessing the unimaginable and not walking away. There is a word for this: allyship. This is what we mean when we say being an ally is so important.

Defined as "an active, consistent, and arduous practice of unlearning and re-evaluating, in which a person in a position of privilege and power seeks to operate in solidarity with a marginalized group,"[99] allyship is one of those words that makes some roll their eyes or sigh as one more politically correct word enters our vocabulary. If we set aside definitions and concepts, however, George Floyd's community showed us exactly how powerful a tool allyship is in fighting for social justice. It means standing by a marginalized group, speaking up for a resident called derogatory names by a patient, stepping in when a colleague is being insensitive or rude to another. Being there for the patient, doctor, nurse, maintenance worker who are mistreated.

In short, allyship is one step beyond looking for the helpers; it is coming forward and being counted as one of them. The power of allyship is one of the great lessons the murder of George Floyd has taught us. Of all the things we can do to help our institutions on their difficult journeys toward Diversity, Equity, and Inclusion, allyship is the one thing we all have at our disposal.

When someone has to look for the helpers, may one of us physicians be there among the allies.

---

99 The Anti-Oppression Network. "Allyship." The Anti-Oppression Network, n.d., https://theantioppressionnetwork.com/allyship/

Trials and Tribulations of Recruiting Black Patients for Cancer Research*

Sarah Marion

I was already in the third week of my internship at Memorial Sloan Kettering Cancer Center. I logged onto RedCap to check the status of my breast cancer survey. Unchanged from the week prior, there were only two responses. Technically, there was only one complete response, as the other participant stopped after page one. I was embarrassed, frankly, by how my expectations of the project vastly overestimated survey participation. I was desperate for data given the program's abstract deadline in a few weeks and I was beginning to doubt the feasibility of my project.

My plan was to investigate barriers to cancer care during the COVID-19 pandemic among Black women in a COVID-19 hotspot. Given known baseline differences in access, quality, and outcomes, my research mentor and I wanted to assess barriers we presumed had been worsened by increased unemployment and delays in screenings and treatment among other consequences of the global pandemic.[100]

100 Marion, Sarah, et al. "The COVID-19 Pandemic Has Intensified Health Equity Disparities Among Black Women With Breast Cancer. We Must Act Now." ASCO Daily News. 25 Aug. 2021, https://dailynews.ascopubs.org/do/covid-19-pandemic-has-intensified-health-equity-disparities-among-black-women-breast.

Radio Silence

To ensure robust enrollment in our survey-based study, I spent weeks reaching out to breast cancer forums on multiple websites, working to gain access to email listservs, joining Facebook groups that required administrator approval, and contacting Black churches in Manhattan with pleas to add the survey link to their newsletter.

Understanding the potential hesitancy folks may have with sharing personal medical concerns, our recruitment materials highlighted survey anonymity and that it was led by a Black woman—me. I included a headshot of myself, as well as an explanation that understanding barriers could allow us to design programs to improve cancer care.

Despite exhaustive efforts to obtain survey responses, I was met with radio silence—only one-and-a-half responses.

As a Black woman who has experience collecting personal stories—I started the podcast "When We Had Cancer" where I interview breast cancer survivors)—I was bemused by the seeming inaccessibility of a group to which I belonged.

Skewed Representation

The problem that I encountered last summer is tied to a larger problem in public health. According to the FDA, Black patients with cancer are underrepresented in clinical research and clinical trials.[101] Skewed representation not only biases evidence-based medicine, which guides clinical decision-making for optimal cancer treatments, but also limits the individual benefits of access to innovative treatments not yet available to the public.

---

101 Javier-DesLoges, Juan et al. "Disparities and trends in the participation of minorities, women, and the elderly in breast, colorectal, lung, and prostate cancer clinical trials." *Cancer.* vol. 128, no. 4, Feb 2022, pp. 770-777. doi: 10.1002/cncr.33991

Several factors may drive poor participation of Black patients. Lack of trust, low health literacy, low socioeconomic status, and decision-making based in spirituality and/or familial opinion are all potential reasons for reduced participation by some.

Physician-related barriers and those caused by structural racism—such as implicit bias, overburdened staff and under-resourced centers—likely also play a role.

Although many studies have explored the reasons for lack of participation, there have been few adequate solutions. Suggested solutions include the integration of educational videos, as well as community-based participatory research strategies, to dispel misconceptions surrounding clinical trials and educate broadly.

While these solutions target lack of trust and some knowledge barriers, they may poorly account for factors such as limited trial availability in treatment facilities or physician bias.

To address financial concerns, which factor more broadly into social determinants of health, honoraria for time spent traveling and participating in clinical research may increase participation. Increased diversity of the physician workforce may both reduce bias within health care and increase trust. Research has shown that Black patients value receiving trial information from someone with the same racial/ethnic identity.

Grassroots Community

Although different from clinical trials and qualitative research studies, the podcast I started in 2019 was successful in recruiting Black women with breast cancer simply through word of mouth.

Through a mutual friend, I was put in contact with the founder of the Thelma D. Jones Breast Cancer Fund. Shortly thereafter, multiple women reached out to participate, presumably feeling more comfortable by an introduction from within a pre-established, supportive grassroots community.

Similar to designated leaders in community-based participatory research, friends and family who informally speak of research studies may ultimately increase trust and clinical research participation. Having current or former Black research volunteers or investigators do outreach may encourage community word of mouth in safe spaces.

Potential venues include Delta Sigma Theta sorority meetups—like those attended by my own parents—recreational/community centers, Black churches, historically Black colleges and universities alumni gatherings, and Black health advocacy groups.

Additional information and talks can be arranged at annual breast cancer walks, including the Race for the Cure and Strides Against Breast Cancer, which are diversely attended and include an activated and enthusiastic audience.

This type of boots-on-the-ground outreach can lay the groundwork for explaining why clinical research matters for Black communities. Myths can be debunked, advantages discussed, and even those potential future participants who are largely swayed by their family's opinions may be accurately informed by parents or children. Fueling participation in clinical trials through word of mouth may be another way to tackle current barriers—engaging communities from within is a key aspect of trust building.

Reflections

By the end of my internship, I switched gears to an entirely new research project evaluating disparities in care for Black women.

Reflecting on research project number one and our failed recruitment strategies, I have become more invigorated than ever to bring the full benefits of scientific advancement into my community and to highlight why clinical research should serve them.

The experience made me realize that this work cannot be accomplished in a research summer; it requires motivated and dedicated physicians, researchers, and community members laying the groundwork for years, investing in communities, forming bonds, and building trust.

As I move forward into my future career as a physician, I hope to do the essential work to bridge this gap. Perhaps in the near future, we can move toward meeting Black women where they are in their communities to approach them for clinical research, instead of expecting them to come to us.

This piece comes from the partnership between the WIMS Blog and the Healio Women in Oncology blog:
Marion, S. Women in Oncology (blog): Trials, tribulations of recruiting Black patients for cancer research. Healio, November 3, 2022. Available at: https://www.wimedicine.org/blog/cancer-patient-research. Reprinted with permission from Healio.

Navigating Health Care as a Physician, Member of LGBTQ+ Community*

BJ Rimel, MD

"Which mom are you?"

It's an innocent question, right? I'm with one of my kids, and I'm alone at their school picking them up. The person asking has never seen me before, but they know we are a queer family.

I invariably reply, "I am the doctor mom."

Of all the identities I could tie to this response, why "doctor mom?" I could be the "taller mom," the "cisgender mom," or the "can't-parallel-park-mom." I could give them what they want upfront and just say, I am the "biological mom." But I never do.

Systemic Barriers

As a medical student in the South in 1999, the vast majority of people I interacted with were kind, rational, and tolerant. I had an occasional disconnect with a patient or doctor who was less than enthusiastic about my completely out approach to my sexual orientation. Most commonly, I was told that I had not met the right man—a role they were offering to play.

In one-on-one interactions, however, most humans gave me a chance to show that I, too, was compassionate, empathetic, and capable. I was mentored. I was offered opportunities to learn, to present, and even to publish research. I got my first choice of residency in the match and again when I applied for fellowship. No doubt, my privilege as a white person played an enormous role in my success. Despite all of these privileges, the systemic barriers I have encountered as a lesbian woman trying to keep my family and spouse safe have taken their toll.

Provider homophobia

Discrimination and fear of discrimination keep many in the sex and gender minority community from seeking health care. A large, systematic review by Ayhan and colleagues describes three main experiences, including discrimination in the health care setting of LGBTQ individuals, the importance of disclosure to providers, and awareness of homophobia and/or transphobia among providers.[102]

The fear of provider homophobia in particular resonates with my lived experience. As a resident in OB/GYN, I knew all about assisted reproduction and even had insurance coverage for infertility. In order to qualify for this, I had to have infertility—hard to prove when your partner doesn't make compatible gametes. But we wanted a family and this was our chance. The physicians in the faculty infertility practice were all skilled. I knew them because I had worked with them on rotations. I chose the one I thought was most likely to be comfortable with me and had other same-sex couples in his practice who the other residents had seen.

---

102 Ayhan CHB, Bilgin H, Uluman OT, Sukut O, Yilmaz S, Buzlu S. A Systematic Review of the Discrimination Against Sexual and Gender Minority in Health Care Settings. *International Journal of Health Services*. 2020;50(1):44-61.

We tried all the usual routes but ended up with in vitro fertilization as our best option in the last month of my residency. At this point, I had matched in St. Louis. We would lose our infertility coverage and, thus, our chance to have a family until we had a different financial situation.

On the night of my graduation dinner, we had our oocyte retrieval. This meant the very last week of my residency would be the transfer. This was before the days of cryopreservation. The practice model was that the on-call doctor would perform the transfer. Of course, not everyone in the practice was comfortable with same-sex couples. One provider refused to treat homosexual couples on religious grounds. If they were the on-call person, would I get the transfer?

The morning of transfer brought the doctor who doesn't treat same-sex-couples. I was certain I would be turned away. I didn't even bother changing into the gown. We looked at each other and he said, "Hi, I'm your doctor for today."

The transfer resulted in a pregnancy. We were thrilled. As I began to show, however, we began to recognize the discriminatory comments that showed how we were often viewed by the system as invalid. At our first ultrasound for anatomy, the technician turned to my wife and said, "When will you have one of your own?" When I was signing in for labor and delivery, I put my wife's name and contact information for my emergency contact and as the baby's second parent. The form had only a space for "father " but I used it anyway. The charge nurse came to me in the waiting area and loudly proclaimed that "the baby's father can't be a woman" and demanded I rewrite the form "properly."

Doctor mom

Our daughter is now 14. The transfer of her embryo was the first of many sleepless nights. There were more, such as when we had a home study in order to adopt our daughter because the state that we lived in made her parentage by two women illegal or the times when my wife was run out of women's bathrooms trying to change her. The insomnia is tempered by finding a queer pediatrician, then a Medicare expansion, and then an EMR upgrade that finally carries my sexual orientation as a discrete variable.

So, I own that "doctor mom" title. I want folks to know we are a queer family, and I am part of a legacy of physicians who are making that intersection stronger.

This piece comes from the partnership between the WIMS Blog and the Healio Women in Oncology blog:

Rimel, BJ. Women in Oncology (blog): Navigating health care as a physician, member of LGBTQ+ community. Healio, October 13, 2022. Available at: https://www.wimedicine.org/blog/physician-lgbtqia-community. Reprinted with permission from Healio.

We Need to Talk About Womxn

Davy Ran, MD, MSc, MPH

Womxn. How do you pronounce that word? In my mind, I say "wo-mix-in", which feels like it gets at the core concept of the word: women, with a few other genders mixed in, but to a lesser extent.

Womxn is a pretty universal signal for attempted inclusion. I have never heard this word used with ill intent. However, I can think of many times that word has made me feel actively uncomfortable and unwelcome as a nonbinary person.

Once, in college, my therapist suggested I try group therapy. "I have a women's group that would be *great* for you," she'd enthused, and it took me several stunned seconds to gather myself enough to remind her:

"I'm ... not a woman."

I watched her eyes go wide in recognition of her error and she stumbled over several apologies before we moved on. At the end of the visit, though, she brought it up again; "You could still attend the women's group, you know. I'm sure no one would have a problem with a nonbinary person joining."

Huh. Well. I was glad that no one *else* would have a problem, but what about *my* problem?

When a cis man is not allowed into a women's-only space, they are validated as being *not a woman*. What does it say to lump trans men, nonbinary folx, and all others* existing under a clearly nonwoman umbrella into women's groups, spaces, and stories? She might as well have said, "You corrected me, but I still see you as a woman, I have decided that *my* consent and comfort is the priority over yours."

To be clear, being AFAB (Assigned Female At Birth) and nonbinary is not a form of *diet woman* or *woman-lite*. Much as women don't want to be defined in relation to men (see, for example, "women doctors" vs "doctors"), other genders should not be defined solely in relation to the genders they are not.

The confusion, I think, comes from trying to reconcile the way the patriarchy oppresses *all* genders besides men with intersectional feminism attempts to empower *all* oppressed genders. Historically, conversations around these two opposing forces have been focused exclusively on cisgender women and men.

As someone who is AFAB and, for much of my life, perceived as a woman by others, I feel a lot of solidarity with women and the truly incessant sexist messaging they and I received growing up. As someone who is non-binary, I feel solidarity with women as another underrecognized, underrepresented, and continually undermined gender, though we are all these things in different ways. These two feelings of solidarity are not the same, nor should they be. When we equivocate women's experiences with the experiences of other genders, we not only erase the unique experiences of other genders but also the unique experiences of women.

At an old workplace, my boss, a man, would habitually make sexual comments, often outfit related, towards women on staff. As someone who dressed more "masculine," these comments were never applied to me. I did, however, get my own share of transphobic commentary, which the cis women did not. We deserved the space to process these feelings and, while we could all agree harassment is wrong, it did not magically make us able to understand the depth of each other's experiences as though we'd experienced them ourselves.

That said, it is not impossible nor inappropriate for women's organizations to aim for inclusion. There are ways it can be done with grace and skill. If one wants to invite trans people who aren't women or woman-aligned into women's spaces, make it clear they are being included, not as add-ons or as a "close enough" to women, but explicitly as *trans people who aren't women* (with their consent, of course!**). Actively recognize the differences in experience and the nuances and benefits of trans voices in gender equity conversations precisely *because* they are trans voices, as opposed to in spite of. We don't need to be the same to deserve the same rights and pursue the same goal.

In being encouraged to write this piece for WIM, I was given the option of raising my voice as whatever identity I wanted to share. By defining itself as an organization for women, allies, and those to whom they are allied, WIM provides a venue in which gender equity can be discussed, dissected, and pursued by all angles by all people. We don't need womxn to do this; we don't need to be afraid of naming more precisely that to which we speak. It may be wordy, but it's worth it. At the risk of sounding cliche, all of us minoritized identities really *are* in this together, and I look forward to continuing the fight for gender equity in the spirit of ever-evolving integration—and *not* assimilation—in the future.

> *There are as many genders as there are people—identities are limitless! Other commonly cited gender identities in American culture include genderqueer, genderfluid, agender, bigender, and Two-Spirit (a Native American identity only).*

> **I cannot emphasize enough how much I do not speak for all trans people, and the best way to know how trans people want to be included is to ask them. Having this option open to people, though, will serve as a better catch-all than 'womxn' does.*

A More Inclusive Medical School Graduation Ceremony

Eileen Barrett, MD, MPH

In 2017, I had the privilege of working with two medical students whose first languages were different from my own; I was raised in an English-speaking home (and only speak English), whereas one of them was raised in a Spanish-speaking home and the other was raised in a Navajo-and English-speaking home. We spoke about what a gift it is to speak several languages, and how important it is to feel like we belong. Having recently read an article about a medical school planning to say the Hippocratic Oath in several languages during graduation, I asked if pursuing something like that locally could help graduation be more inclusive, and they both said yes.

When I was on faculty at the University of New Mexico, graduating students recited the Physician's Pledge that is maintained by the World Medical Association (WMA).[103] The WMA has long had the Physician's Pledge available in French, Spanish, and English; in

---

103 Parsa-Parsi, Ramin Walter. "The Revised Declaration of Geneva: A Modern-Day Physician's Pledge." *Journal of the American Medical Association*. vol. 318, no. 20, Nov. 2017, pp. 1971-1972. doi: 10.1001/jama.2017.16230

more recent years, it was translated into multiple other languages—but not yet to Navajo. To try to get this translated into Navajo (and then advocate for adoption by the WMA), a colleague connected me with Mr. Frank Morgan who is a senior, bilingual, Navajo educator affiliated with Diné College. Mr. Morgan graciously supported moving forward with this effort and quickly provided a culturally relevant translation and interpretation he had produced.

After receiving a copy of Mr. Morgan's translation, I shared it with the WMA and requested it be accepted as an official translation. After several months' time, follow up, and explanations, the Navajo language interpretation of the Pledge was officially adopted, with Mr. Morgan receiving the credit he is due.[104] Soon afterward, I approached the medical school, where I was faculty, to ask if the Navajo and Spanish language versions of the Pledge could be included in graduation. I cited how this is relevant to our patients, learners, and staff and could help us be more inclusive of New Mexicans in general. Unfortunately, leadership didn't agree this should happen and cited that graduation could be too long if others wanted their first languages represented.

I was profoundly disappointed when I heard the decision. Fortunately, my husband (and my biggest supporter) recommended I not give up and that I build a team that can double down on educating the senior leadership on the experiences of our learners from Spanish-speaking and Navajo-speaking communities. A senior leader in DEI supported this idea, offered her support, and recommended I reconnect with the students who inspired the work. I was embarrassed I hadn't done this the first time, as I had made the

---

104 World Medical Association. Navajo Declaration of Geneva. World Medical Association, Mar. 2018, https://www.wma.net/wp-content/uploads/2018/10/Navajo_Declaration-of-Geneva-3_26_18.pdf.

wrong assumption that adopting this would be an obvious positive change to graduation.

Connecting with those students was inspiring. They led the charge thereafter, speaking with senior leaders in multiple venues. Their work culminated in the Physician's Pledge being read in English, Spanish, and Navajo during graduation starting in 2019 and every year since. Since then, I've collaborated with a now-former resident on getting the Pledge translated into Arabic, and I'm now working with a leader in Zuni Pueblo to translate it into the Zuni language (another Indigenous language in our state).

It is a minor but meaningful change to medical school graduation to include content such as saying the Physician's Pledge in the languages spoken by students. While this may not seem like explicit gender equity work, women can and absolutely should continue to participate in this type of advocacy work. For me, this was brought home when one former student who orchestrated pledge efforts led its recitation during graduation in 2019. It was reinforced just last month when the other student who helped inspire this work told me the only part of any of her graduations her mother has ever understood was the Pledge recital in Spanish at her medical school graduation in 2019.

Out of the Closet and into the Conference

Davy Ran, MD, MSc, MPH

When I think about the phrase coming out, I think about a teenager sitting their parents down in a living room and saying "Mom, Dad, I think I'm gay." I don't think about a twenty-eight-year-old medical student who's been out as queer for over a decade realizing only as they stand to present a conference that no one listening knows their pronouns.

Which is why, of course, that's the exact situation I found myself in at the most recent conference I attended; I was handed a badge containing neither the name nor pronouns I actually go by. The conference staff were exceedingly kind and immediately offered to reprint my tag, but when they asked me what to put on it, I hesitated.

"Just put Davy," I said after a moment, fidgeting with my poster. "No pronouns, it's fine."

How do we, as trans people, navigate the hovering potential of transphobia in professional spaces, especially transient ones? This was just one of many little moments of discomfort I often experience at work events as a nonbinary person using they/them pronouns, less the result of any individual actions and more the result of overarching sociocultural transphobia.

As a high-energy extrovert, I've introduced myself to hundreds of people at conferences over the years. After four years of conference-going, I still struggle to ascertain how out I should be during these introductions. In so many spaces, being openly trans can be actively dangerous, and it is impossible to know at first glance what kind of space a work conference holds. Even at LGBT-themed conferences in the heart of queer neighborhoods, many people do not know what non-binary is or how to consciously use they/them pronouns. So I never know, when introducing myself, what level of queer cultural knowledge and competency people are at and how they feel about it.

With every person I meet I wonder, will I . . .

- Be safe in coming out?
- Need to educate about my identity?
- Need to defend my openness about my identity?
- Ruin my conference experience?
- Risk my future career?

I am lucky to be proudly and delightedly out in all areas of my life, as anyone who looks me up will know. That said, outness is an ongoing journey requiring constant upkeep, especially if one is continually meeting new people. Do I have the time and energy to explain/defend/justify my identity over several days to hundreds of people who I may never see again, while trying to attend and learn and present at a work conference simultaneously?

Lately, the answer for me has been *No*. It's a hefty demand on top of the regular demands of medical school. As a medical student attending conferences, I work hard to stay in the student role, and the switch to educator is not as easy as it sounds. It is *hard* to be the only person in the room introducing their pronouns. It is *hard* to teach many people you don't know—kindly, patiently, and effectively—what pronouns are during a sixty-second introduction. It is hard to interrupt conversations with constant reminders of my pronouns and to extensively comfort those who mess up. And although it is energy-draining to be misgendered unknowingly, it's not nearly so draining as to be misgendered knowingly.

Ultimately, the most effective short-term way I have found to avoid transphobia is to simply pretend I don't exist, to simply pretend that I am cis, until asked or proven otherwise.

It's not ideal, and it's not forever. As more conferences add things like chosen names and pronouns to IDs, queer and trans flag badges for attendees to wear, education and emphasis on inclusive greetings, openly transgender staff and speakers, and workshops and lectures on the transgender community, cultural competency is becoming more commonplace, accepted, and in some places required.

At this most recent conference full of wonderful allies, I saw one person label their ID with pronouns. That person was not me. But that person *did* prompt others to bring up their pronouns, which made me more comfortable mentioning my own.

In the end, whether or not I choose to out myself at work conferences depends entirely on how quick, easy, and safe it is to do so. Clear cultural competency signaling from all of us is crucial to create conferences that are educational, inclusive, and empowering for all. I look forward to building this space together!

Is It Really a "Leaky Pipeline" If We Are Actively Pushing People Out?*

Evanie Anglade, BA

I am a Black physician in training, and at times, I feel like I may lose my spot.

In 2015, Black residents accounted for approximately 5% of all residents, yet they accounted for almost 20% of those who were dismissed, according to reporting by the Accreditation Council for Graduate Medical Education.[105,106]

Underrepresented minority (URM) individuals attempting to pursue a career in medicine are exiting the "leaky pipeline" (a visual image that represents how many moments and changes exist for underrepresented individuals to fall off professional development pathways) at many time-points on the medicine journey (from the

---

105 Accreditation Council for Graduate Medical Education. Diversity and inclusion in graduate medical education. Accreditation Council for Graduate Medical Education, 2019, https://southernhospitalmedicine.org/wp-content/uploads/2019/10/McDade-ACGME-SHM-Presentation-McDade-Final.pdf.
106 Association of American Medical Colleges. Diversity in Medicine: Facts and Figures 2019. Association of American Medical Colleges, 2019, https://www.aamc.org/data-reports/workforce/report/diversity-medicine-facts-and-figures-2019.

college pre-med track, medical school, residency, fellowship, and beyond) at disproportionately higher rates compared with their counterparts.

Unexpected Departures

Within my own experience, I can reflect on times when it felt like fellow URM trainees were unfairly targeted and had unexpected departures under obscure circumstances.

While working as a medical scribe, I can recall overhearing hospital staff discussing how the only Black orthopedic resident at the time was let go—yet another URM resident they had seen who was mysteriously dismissed from their program.

Even just a few weeks ago, the former Chief Diversity Officer at University Hospital resigned, later recounting her experience of feeling targeted, demeaned, and disrespected as a Black female physician in a leadership position.[107]

The issue with the "leaky pipeline" analogy is that it describes the phenomenon as a passive occurrence—as if it were bound to happen without external influences. Prior research and my own lived experience would indicate that this is simply not the case; often, obstacles forcing URM individuals out of the workforce are factors outside of their control.

Deficits in educational and sponsorship opportunities and elements of both structural racism and microaggression stop qualified and motivated URM individuals from advancing further along the medicine journey, especially when securing positions of leadership.

---

107 Llorente, Elizabeth. "Racism pervades this N.J. hospital, former exec says. She was forced out because of it, she claims." NJ.com. 15 Dec. 2022, https://www.nj.com/healthfit/2022/09/racism-pervades-this-nj-hospital-former-exec-says-she-was-forced-out-because-of-it-she-claims.html

Pervasive Disparities

We are seeing that racial and ethnic disparities are pervasive in the physician workforce, as the racial and ethnic demography of the active physician workforce in 2019 did not reflect that of the US population in the 2020 Census.[108]

Less is known about the racial and ethnic representation in leadership, especially within oncology. Our team has previously published about disparities in NCI-Designated Cancer Center leadership in *JAMA Network Open* and wanted to better understand the diversity of teams who created national cancer guidelines.[109]

This summer, I worked to evaluate the National Comprehensive Cancer Network and found, unsurprisingly, that significant racial and ethnic disparities exist, with disproportionately white and Asian committee members compared with both the US Census and active physician workforce.

Even committees creating guidelines for the deadliest cancers in Black and Hispanic patients were not more likely to have Black and Hispanic members—some committees did not have a single Black or Hispanic member. This work serves as important baseline data, which I hope to see improve over my career as I enter residency, fellowship, and, ultimately, the physician workforce.

Personal Path

My work with Dr. Chino encouraged me to reflect upon my own experiences as a Black woman navigating the path into medicine.

108 United States Census Bureau. "Quick Facts." United States Census Bureau. 28 Sep. 2022, https://www.census.gov/quickfacts/fact/table/US/PST045221.

109 Morgan, Austin et al. "Racial, Ethnic, and Gender Representation in Leadership Positions at National Cancer Institute-Designated Cancer Centers." *Journal of the American Medical Association.* vol. 4, no. 6,2021 Jun. 1, :e2112807. pp. 10.1001/jamanetworkopen.2021.12807

Mentorship has gotten me to where I am today—it opened doors and provided me with opportunities to demonstrate my merit. Many of these pivotal mentorship experiences were possible through programs and initiatives dedicated to supporting URM students.

In college, I participated in the Summer Undergraduate Minority Research Program at the University of Pennsylvania in which I was paired with two research mentors, both anesthesiologists, who took me under their wing to learn about their field and conduct health services research. This was my first introduction into clinical medicine and the rewards of research. I continued working with one of my mentors throughout college and into my postgrad years. This experience served to be a key highlight on my medical school application, helping me secure a place at Rutgers' New Jersey Medical School (NJMS).

While at NJMS, I joined my school's Student National Medical Association (SNMA) chapter and was matched with a student mentor who had previously participated in the Memorial Sloan Kettering Cancer Center Summer Pipeline Program. My student mentor encouraged me to apply and ultimately connected me with Dr. Chino. The Pipeline Program provides funding and a research mentor to URM students, and it helped me with resources and opportunities to support my success in medicine. Overall, my experience thus far has shown me that pipeline programs can help provide opportunities to students like me to navigate both the academic and hidden curricula of medicine.

Opportunity began before I even started medical school, however. I think about where I would be today had my parents, both Haitian immigrants, not made the calculated decision and immense effort to move our family to a better-resourced area with greater access to social, economic, and educational opportunities. They understood the impact of one's environment on their future ability to succeed. Because of their sacrifice, I was able to attend well-funded public schools, take SAT prep courses, get into an Ivy League university and, ultimately, get accepted into medical school.

Growing up, I did not fully realize the significance and impact of my parents' efforts. I did not see them as the registered nurse with an hourly wage and the self-employed cab driver who worked tirelessly to keep up with mortgage payments and steep property taxes to allow my siblings and me to attend the good schools we did. I now see that if it were not for my parents' efforts, I may not have found the audacity to pursue a career as a physician.

Everyone Should be Involved

With all the opportunity that has been bestowed, I have made it my mission to serve as a resource to those like me who are also interested in a career in medicine. I have mentored high school students interested in STEM, pre-med, and college, as well as graduate-level URM women applying to medical school. In addition I currently serve as SNMA co-president and mentor first-year medical students. I have used my experiences (both successes and failures) to help these students achieve their goals and offer encouragement, ensuring they know that they, too, have a place in the medical field.

Patching the pipeline should not only be the responsibility of those it affects. Everyone should be involved for the betterment of society and to best care for patients. Those in positions of power need to advocate for holistic review of applications for both trainees and hires, offer admissions and hiring committee seats to diverse staff (and reward these efforts), increase funding for enrichment opportunities catered to URM individuals (like those programs that benefited me), and seek to actively educate themselves and diversify their ranks.

Unfortunately, there is always a looming fear I could be lost from this "leaky pipeline" like so many other promising Black medical trainees. I have realized that my merit and my parents' investment may still not be enough to propel me forward and allow me to succeed when pervasive societal ills continue to foster unequal footing and discrimination. After all, all it takes is one biased senior faculty member to spike my career, especially if there are no supportive people in positions of power to defend me.

My hope is that, through all our collective efforts to change the status quo and support URM trainees, we will be able to make the "leaky pipeline" a phenomenon of the past.

This piece comes from the partnership between the WIMS Blog and the Healio Women in Oncology blog:

Anglade, E. Women in Oncology (blog): Is it really a "leaky pipeline" if we are actively pushing people out? Healio, October 5, 2022. Available at: https://www.wimedicine.org/blog/leaky-pipeline. Reprinted with permission from Healio.

My Brown Woman Doctor White Coat

Rida Khan, MD

Recently, after graduating from medical school and completing my last board exam, Step 3, I decided to branch out and indulge in forgotten joys, things I used to like that may have dampened over the past few coming-of-age years. I reached out to several professional organizations of which I was a student member and volunteered to join the newsletter, more to edit and organize than to write. I have not written in a while (apart from sporadic diaries, Tweets, and Tumblr posts—my roommate in college told me those don't count), and as a constitutionally shy person, I wouldn't put myself out there for the world. Everyone was very excited to have me on board. One of the editors told me enthusiastically that I would have a unique perspective for their publication, as a female medical student during the COVID pandemic. Feebly and stupidly, I said, "I don't know if I'll have anything to say about it other than that it was horrible and I hated it," and flashed a wide and anxious smile.

That moment is etched into my memory: the tone of my voice, the expression I wore, the instant censure of the super-ego setting in microseconds later. The minute I expressed my truth, I felt inadequate and like the embodiment of a massive disappointment. While I am still deciphering the mystery of that exchange, I am coming to see that the world desires us to capitalize on our strengths and weaknesses in equal measure—which is to say that strengths and weaknesses are relative, fluid definitions of phenomena, far from set in stone. A weakness is not a weakness at all.

The truth is that when COVID hit, I was in my penultimate year of medical school, and it struck me with an impossible case of Imposter Syndrome. For over three years prior, I had been waking up every morning to go to the hospital, spending days full of exhilaration, action, and an exuberant diversity of people, and coming back late and exhausted in the best way possible.

We were in our cardiology rotation when COVID struck and the world shut down; I had been excited for the series of lectures we were to have on congenital heart diseases, a convoluted subject that, regardless of its staunchly anatomical basis, requires considerable detective work; the lectures were to be delivered by leading clinicians, contextualized and peppered with clinical insight unavailable in any textbook or paper—exactly my jam. I had been preparing for my Step 2 CK exam to be taken two weeks later, which became "postponed indefinitely" overnight. And my hard-earned summer subinternship in inpatient psychiatry was knocked over like ninepins. All happened in a matter of days.

This would have been prime time for me to sit back and meditate, a practice I learned many years prior, but I was on top of my game at the time, and it took a while to internalize how drastically the world was changing all around. Compounded with all the large-scale problems that COVID began to unearth, from health care inequalities to surges in domestic violence as everyone stayed at home, it would have been a Herculean feat to sit back and take a deep breath at any moment, but I did it. Finally, I did it. I wondered what took so long.

The truth is that being a girl in society shaped every aspect of my life and carried over into my womanhood. I was a stoic female child, pre-adolescent, adolescent, and young adult. I was strong, willful, and driven. I was so busy doing things all the time that I did not realize that I was hurtling through life and not adopting a narrative that was so important to have; by that time, I was living a very specific life—that of a woman, in a developed nation, brown, an immigrant, in medical school, first physician in the family. Taken all together, it sounds quite sensational and ticks all the requirements for a good story. But I hadn't even internalized the fact that I was a medical student yet, and I was soon to be called a doctor? I was so busy living the story of my life, I didn't realize there were lessons all around to be learned and exchanged.

Lately, I have been meditating and rediscovering hidden strengths. Carpe diem. The other day, I went to the beach and walked my legs into the waves, up to my knees. From nowhere, or perhaps from the salty smell of the sea or the rush of the waves or the orange blob of sun setting on the horizon came the memories of how my body would be policed as a girl, what clothes were declared ladylike enough to wear and which weren't, how high you could roll up your jeans so the tide wouldn't get you below the knees. The thought sprung to me: how growing up a girl molded my developing brain in ways I would have had otherwise, had it been my prerogative.

Time to make it my prerogative and start by telling a story. Time to put on your brown girl suit. Time to put on your brown woman doctor white coat. After all, it's the only one that fits.

The Stigma of Being a Caribbean Medical Student

Jessica Rebaza, MS, CHES

The stigma of being a Caribbean medical student can be crippling in many ways. It is so intense that I even fed into it when I was a premed student. I used to believe that going to medical school in the Caribbean was for undisciplined students who didn't work hard enough, for students who didn't have what it took to make it. It wasn't until I became a Caribbean medical student that I realized that the stigma was based on fear, doubt, and lack of knowledge.

My story of becoming a medical student is nontraditional, yet extraordinarily common in many ways in Caribbean medical schools. As a first-generation future doctor, I entered college naively. I didn't know much about what it took to become a physician aside from what I saw on TV. I knew I had to take science classes and the MCAT and submit my application. I figured that couldn't be too hard until I entered chemistry class and struggled immensely. While I did decently in physics and biology, my chemistry classes held me back. I took the MCAT and struggled to score well. I attempted the exam multiple times until I was finally at a national average. Aside from that, my CV from college was packed to the rim—Latinx ambassador for the University of Georgia, president and founder of a medical association in college, medical brigade participant, Spanish translator, shadow of many physicians, and hospital volunteer.

After I graduated from college, I applied to medical school and was rejected without even a chance to interview. I was dedicated to becoming a physician so I worked on my application flaws. I retook the undergraduate chemistry classes that held me back and started my master's degree at Columbia University. I also worked full-time as a nutritionist for two years and interned at the NYC Department of Health and Mental Hygiene. I reapplied to medical school and was able to secure one interview. Once again, I got rejected. I had spent nine years trying to get into medical school by this point. My entire academic and professional career was geared towards one goal, and I had failed to meet it. I was at a complete loss in life until I turned to my last resource—going to medical school abroad.

Even as I applied, interviewed, and attended orientation, my mind was flooded with the thought of the stigma of attending a Caribbean medical school. In my head, I thought of comments that were said to me, such as:

- *If you're as good as you say you are, why aren't you in an American school?*
- *You're going to fail out.*
- *You'll never match into residency.*

However, as I got to know my classmates, I realized that we were all far from failures. Almost every student I met in my first-year class had attended some of the best universities in the United

States, including UCLA, UMiami, UMinnesota, UFlorida, UPenn, UC-Berkeley, Georgetown, Ohio State University, Rutgers, Michigan State, UConn, and Cornell. Most of them also had master's degrees in biochemistry, medical sciences, or public health. Unfortunately, these students were part of the 50-60% of premed students who are not accepted to an American medical school each year. Students, just like me, who worked extremely hard but were overlooked.

Currently, I'm in my second year of medical school and will soon be done with all my preclinical classes. This summer, I will be eligible to sit for the USMLE and I'll begin third-year rotations in the fall. Before I know it, I'll be sending in my application for residency. In the end, attending a Caribbean medical school has allowed me to open a door that had been closed for a very long time. Given everything I've been through in the last eleven years, there shouldn't be any shame or stigma around the fact that I did everything in my power to one day become a physician. From my first day of college to now, I have grown into a professional who doesn't buckle when faced with rejection or failure. If younger me could see me now, she'd be proud of the woman I've become, and she'd thank me for never giving up.

Increasing the Visibility of Peruvian Women Physicians

Jessica Rebaza, MS, CHES

Like many first-generation students, I am the first in my family to attend medical school. Being the first means treading through uncharted territory, which can be intimidating and lonely. Stepping into spaces where there are not people who are similar to you often means you have limited, if any, role models. As a Latina of Peruvian and Puerto Rican descent, I have never met a woman physician of either descent. However, I was aware of the legacy of outstanding Puerto Rican women physicians, such as Drs. Antonia Novello and Helen Rodríguez Trías to name a few. Learning about their contributions to medicine and their leadership has inspired me to know that I, too, can achieve great things in the field. But where were the stories of Peruvian women physicians? Half of my identity seemed to be invisible in medicine.

While the Latin community supports one another regardless of nationality, we are not a monolith. Thus, having subcultures represented in medicine can increase the drive for more women of various Latin descents to step into the medical field. In the

United States, only 5.8% of physicians identify as Hispanic/Latino. A further breakdown shows that only 40% of Latin physicians are women.[110] Besides that, we don't know these women's cultures or backgrounds. Are they of Mexican, Ecuadorian or Cuban descent? Are they of mixed descent like me?

With this curiosity of finding more Peruvian women physicians, I took to Twitter. I wrote, *"Growing up half-Peruvian, I have never met a Peruvian woman doctor. Please share your favorite Peruvian women physicians with me."*[111] In all honesty, I did not expect it to go anywhere. After all, I spent twenty-eight years of life without ever meeting a single Peruvian physician, yet alone a Peruvian woman physician. But, to my surprise, my tweet blew up overnight with over a hundred likes and 42 responses from Peruvian women physicians from all over the country. I beamed with pride. All of the parts that make me who I am today—my language, foods, culture, music, and experiences—were finally coming together. I could now fully see myself represented holistically in medicine.

Even being Latina, I had to search for others, which means there is not enough visibility for Latina physicians and less for Peruvian women physicians. However, I learned from that tweet that there are organizations that support this initiative, including the Peruvian American Medical Society (PAMS) and the social-media based Peruvian Physicians Training in the US. In addition, I learned of Dr. Bertha Bouroncle, who discovered hairy cell leukemia in

---

110 American Association of Medical Colleges. Diversity in Medicine: Facts and Figures 2019. American Association of Medical Colleges, 2019, https://www.aamc.org/data-reports/workforce/report/diversity-medicine-facts-and-figures-2019.

111 Jessica Rebaza, MS [@JessicaRebaza]. "Growing up Half Peruvian, I Have Never Met a Peruvian Woman Doctor. Please Share Your Favorite Peruvian Women Physicians with Me! @Latinasinmed @Wimsummit #Latinxmedtwitter #Medtwitter #Latinxinmedicine #Womeninmedicine #Peruvian #Peru." Twitter, 5 June 2021, https://twitter.com/themedicaledit/status/1401220002485841929.

1958 and also happens to be from my family's town. I also connected with Peruvian women physicians in all fields of medicine who have become my new role models for what a life in medicine looks like for someone of my cultural background.

To continue to increase the visibility, I've done my small part in becoming a member of PAMS and adding the Peruvian flag emoji to my social media profiles. That alone has inspired Peruvian women premedical students to reach out to say that they're motivated to continue their career in medicine because they know they're not alone. This visibility is not only important for Peruvian women but for women of all cultural and ethnic backgrounds. By sharing the stories and uplifting the voices of these women, we can help the next generation of women leaders in medicine.

Chapter 12

ABORTION AND WOMEN'S HEALTH

"With Sorrow"

Avital O'Glasser, MD, FACP, SFHM, DFPM

With sorrow—for this Court, but more,
for the many millions of American women who have today lost a
fundamental constitutional protection—we dissent.
—JUSTICES STEPHEN BREYER, SONIA SOTOMAYOR AND ELENA KAGAN,
JUNE 24TH, 2022[112]

With the Friday, June 24, 2022, Supreme Court majority opinion overturning *Roe v. Wade*, five decades of protection for reproductive rights came crashing down. With dozens of states awaiting this decision, with dozens of states passing or planning abortion bans or severe restrictions, the landscape of access to safe abortions in this country is scarred and destroyed.

With sorrow

This—in a country that already has horrendous maternal and childhood mortality rates. In a country without universal health-care. In a country with a political faction that proclaims they are "pro-life" but do not support paid family leave, access to desper-

---

112 Dobbs v. Jackson Women's Health Organization, 597 U. S. ___ (2022)

ately needed formula, anti-racist or anti-homophobic policies, or life-saving gender affirming care. In a country where a vocal contingent so loudly proclaims "my body, my rights" about vaccines, masks, or COVID precautions—but does not respect or protect a woman's right to choose regarding "HER body, HER rights." In a country where a gun has more freedom and rights than a woman. In a country, where at least until today, "respecting a woman as an autonomous being, and granting her full equality, meant giving her substantial choice over this most personal and most consequential of all life decisions."[113]

With sorrow
Women will die. People with uteruses will die. Women will lose the reproductive freedom that is protected by access to safe abortion, which itself protects access to education, professional development, future income potential, financial security, and the opportunity to build generational wealth—as well as access to protection from domestic and intimate partner violence. Women will also lose access to abortion following rape, incest, tragic prenatal diagnoses, and life-threatening pregnancy complications. Women who lose access to abortion "will incur the cost of losing control of their lives."[114] And, in another sick, paradoxical twist, abortion bans may prevent access to IVF and fertility treatment.

With sorrow
And it won't end with abortion. In a concurring opinion, Justice Thomas wrote, "we should reconsider all of this Court's substantive due process precedents, including Griswold, Lawrence,

---

113 ibid.
114 ibid.

and Obergefell."[115] If you haven't been paying attention, those are the cases that protect contraception, same-sex relationships, and same-sex marriage. Even the dissenting justices have issued their Cassandra cry: "No one should be confident that this majority is done with its work. The right Roe and Casey recognized does not stand alone."[116] What other personal liberties and rights—especially for the most vulnerable amongst us—are at risk?

So, with sorrow, we shed our tears, beat our breasts, wail our laments. With sorrow, we say, *"we told you this would happen!"* in 2016, and with every up-ticket and down-ticket election since then. With sorrow, we hug our daughters, text our friends, and try to keep moving through the day. With sorrow, we think of those harmed today, tomorrow, and in the years to come. And with sorrow, we plan our rage, activism, and advocacy—and how we will fight to protect our rights and our safety.

Because, with sorrow, we know that today's Supreme Court decision will not end abortion in this country, but it may very well end access to *safe* abortion in this country.

Because, with sorrow, we know that the attack on our rights does not end today—but neither does the fight to protect them.

Because, with sorrow, we band together to strengthen our reserve and our resolve.

Because—with sorrow—we dissent.

---

115 ibid.
116 ibid.

Healthcare Crisis

Grace Keegan, MS; Julie Chor, MD, MPH

As medical professionals, we are committed to helping our patients achieve their full health potential and cannot be silent as our patients experience forced pregnancy. While the final Supreme Court *Dobbs v. Jackson Women's Health Organization* decision *overturning Roe v. Wade* will have many tragic consequences for our patients, it will also inflict a moral injury on medical trainees and providers who will live and practice in states where they will be legally restricted from providing essential medical care.

The Court's Dobbs decision will have substantial implications on medical training, which will in turn only worsen existing health inequities. The case will limit where future doctors may receive the training necessary to provide essential healthcare to people who could become pregnant. Additionally, with this ruling we have lost the right to uphold our patients' dignity, bodily autonomy, and reproductive freedom in our medical practice. Limitations on abortion training will also impact education and training surrounding contraception, miscarriage management, and ectopic pregnancy management. Educational training for abortion care is imperative to ensure continued capacity to provide the full spectrum of reproductive healthcare.

States will be able to impose restrictions on medical education and training related to providing abortion care and counseling; consequently, the already small number of residency training programs that offer family planning rotations will drop in many states in the coming year.[117] Given that one in four people who can become pregnant in the US has an abortion in their lifetime,[118] and that abortion bans do not reduce the number of people needing abortion services,[119] abortion restrictions will leave tens of thousands of people seeking these essential services with few places to turn for care. Doctors and trainees who live in states that uphold *their* right to provide abortion care are already becoming inundated with requests from people seeking this care from other states. Such overwhelmed systems will almost certainly lead to poorer health outcomes for patients and moral distress for medical trainees and providers.

As healthcare providers, we are trained to uphold the ethical principle of "beneficence," or to act for the ultimate benefit of the patient above all. As a medical student (GK), I am compelled to seek further medical training only in states that will allow me to uphold these commitments. As a medical educator, I (JC) am compelled to advise students to train in states that will prepare them to provide comprehensive reproductive healthcare, which includes abortion care.

---

117 Herbitter, Cara et al. " Family planning training in US family medicine residencies." *Family Medicine*. vol. 43, no. 8, Sep. 2011, pp. 574-81.

118 Jones, Rachel K. and Jenna Jerman. "Population Group Abortion Rates and Lifetime Incidence of Abortion: United States, 2008-2014." *American Journal of Public Health*. vol. 107, no. 12, Dec. 2017, pp. 1904-1909. doi: 10.2105/AJPH.2017.304042.

119 Bearak, Jonathan et al. "Unintended pregnancy and abortion by income, region, and the legal status of abortion: estimates from a comprehensive model for 1990-2019." *The Lancet Global Health*. vol. 8, no. 9, Sep. 2020, e1152-e1161. doi: 10.1016/S2214-109X(20)30315-6

Accordingly, we cannot justify pursuing or recommending training in a state whose laws prevent doctors from making decisions or providing services they feel are in the best interest of patients.

We are not alone in these beliefs with regard to medical training. Medical students are already expressing their intentions to avoid residency training in states banning access to abortion care and training. Many states that have or are expected to ban abortion already have less access to obstetric care and higher rates of maternal mortality.[120] The reversal of Roe will only exacerbate this problem of access to care in the coming years if we do not reaffirm the right to abortion in every state.

Currently 47% of OBGYNs practice in states where they completed residency training.[121] Anticipating that fewer medical students will seek residency training in states without access to abortion training and care, abortion restrictions may have downstream effects on the availability of OBGYNs in these states. Therefore, in addition to immediate repercussions on access to essential reproductive healthcare, our country must recognize that one potentially unforeseen consequence of the decision to overturn *Roe v. Wade* also includes the loss of well-trained future physicians in states with the greatest health challenges.

Our privilege as medical students and providers is that we will likely always have the resources to obtain an abortion, should we

120 United Health Foundation. 2018 Annual Report: Healthiest States. United Health Foundation, 2018, https://www.americashealthrankings.org/learn/reports/2018-annual-report/findings-state-rankings.

121 American Association of Medical Colleges. Active Physicians Practicing in the State Where They Completed Graduate Medical Education (GME) by Specialty, 2019. American Association of Medical Colleges, 2019, https://www.aamc.org/data-reports/workforce/interactive-data/active-physicians-practicing-state-where-they-completed-graduate-medical-education-gme-specialty.

need this care. However, we must speak out as healthcare professionals, knowing that our most vulnerable patients will be disproportionately affected by the Supreme Court's ruling.

The United States has the highest maternal mortality rate among developed countries[122]; it fails to provide universal healthcare, childcare, or paid family leave, and lacks equitable access to contraception.[123] Due to structural barriers to equitable healthcare, those at greatest risk of being impacted by the overturning of Roe are also at a higher risk of experiencing negative health outcomes in pregnancy,[124] outcomes which include complication and death rates that far exceed these risks for legal abortions.[125] In the states that have already passed laws to ban abortion, and those that will do so in the coming days and months, the loss of this previously guaranteed right will cause immeasurable harms to these patients and their families. Put simply, forced pregnancy is not only a violation of fundamental freedoms; it presents a threat to many people's lives.

Given the profound medical, social, and economic consequences prescribed by our country for having a child, abortion is essential health care. Accordingly, medical professionals and trainees have an ethical and professional responsibility to advocate for

---

122 Tikkanen, Roosa et al. Maternal Mortality and Maternity Care in the United States Compared to 10 Other Developed Countries. The Commonwealth Fund, 18 Nov. 2020, https://www.commonwealthfund.org/publications/issue-briefs/2020/nov/maternal-mortality-maternity-care-us-compared-10-countries.

123 Kreitzer, Rebecca J. et al. "Affordable but Inaccessible? Contraception Deserts in the US States." *Journal of Health Policy, Politics, and Law.* vol. 46, no. 2, Apr. 2021, pp. 277-304. doi: 10.1215/03616878-8802186

124 Hoyert, Donna L. Maternal Mortality Rates in the United States, 2020. Centers for Disease Control and Prevention, Feb. 2022, https://www.cdc.gov/nchs/data/hestat/maternal-mortality/2020/maternal-mortality-rates-2020.htm.

125 Kortsmit, Katherine et al. Abortion Surveillance - United States, 2019. Centers for Disease Control and Prevention, 24 Nov. 2021, https://www.cdc.gov/mmwr/volumes/70/ss/ss7009a1.htm.

expanded access to abortion care for our patients and training for our current and future colleagues. Anything short of these goals will undoubtedly lead to devastating outcomes for patients and healthcare professionals alike.

How Do I Ask about Abortion during Match 2023? Reflections from Two Twitter Chats

Abigail Liberty, MD, MSPH; Ian Fields, MD MCR

Match 2023 applications have been submitted, signals designated, and students are awaiting interviews. Given that thirteen states have near-total bans on abortion with elements criminalizing referring for abortion care, residency and medical school applicants are anxious about how restrictions impact education and training. Two social media events sought to create space to speak about these concerns. We'd like to highlight the themes of the chats to empower women in medicine to continue the conversation across all specialties.

The Alliance for Clinical Education hosts a bimonthly chat (#MedEdChat) focused on interdisciplinary and collaborative discussion among preclinical medical educators. On August 18, 2022, @MedEdChat hosted a TwitterChat about abortion restrictions and medical education.

Participants hypothesized that applicants will prioritize training in states without restrictions in order to maximize training opportunities and protect personal bodily autonomy. This is projected to exacerbate competitiveness between states that protect abortion care and those that prohibit it. However, applicants may not forgo a spot in medical school or residency even if they are disappointed to train in a restrictive environment. Current studies are underway by Dr. Vinny Arora, a hospitalist and Dean for Medical Education at the University of Chicago, to understand how restrictions impact applicants' career goals from residency to independent practice. No studies appear available at the medical school application and matriculation level.

Participants reported that no-questions-asked, unlimited and private medical leave is critical for protecting trainees' access to abortion care. Students need proactive guidance navigating insurance and medical systems as adults, and abortion cannot be a blind spot—unaddressed until an acute need arises and a student realizes their insurance does not cover reproductive health. This needs to be actively incorporated into recruitment and onboarding. Participants hypothesized that lack of attention to reproductive health will only exacerbate inequities among medical students and is directly counterproductive to efforts to fortify diversity and inclusion in medicine.

A week following the #MedEdChat, @Inside_TheMatch and OHSU School of Medicine (via @OHSUSOM) co-hosted a chat entitled #AskAboutAbortion to crowdsource advice for residency applicants concerned for the impact of abortion restrictions on their training. The majority of participants included attending physicians, predominantly from the host institution, but with key voices from states with restrictions including Texas and Georgia. Despite nonspecialty specific advertising and the fact that restrictions on reproductive rights have the ability to impact trainees in all specialties, the majority of attendants were OBGYNs or Family Medicine providers.

The discussion voiced concern for deficits in training without abortion care and debated whether experience managing perinatal loss is enough to gain proficiency in those skills. Generally, physicians felt that skills of miscarriage management improve when taught alongside abortion care.[126]

Applicants were encouraged to ask directly about abortion care opportunities if they felt that attending a program that was not supportive of abortion care would be harmful for them. Some applicants reported concern about potential negative ramifications of asking about a controversial topic, namely the fear of discrimination from an interviewer who is anti-abortion. In these situations, physician participants validated that fear and encouraged applicants to ask about adjacent topics: contraception, miscarriage, referrals within the catchment, initiatives aimed at diversity, inclusion and anti-racism. Furthermore, people shared that in their experience, trainees who do not intend to provide abortion care are also disadvantaged by policies which stigmatize or abortion care.

Lastly, the chat discussed the specifics about the importance of national curriculum objectives in advocating for abortion care. The ACGME accreditation guidelines for OBGYN education were addended to prevent discrediting of programs now barred from providing abortion care and to provide a framework to ensure

---

126 Freedman, Lori R. et al. "When there's a heartbeat: miscarriage management in Catholic-owned hospitals." *American Journal of Public Health.* vol. 98, no. 10, Oct. 2008, pp. 1774-8. doi: 10.2105/AJPH.2007.126730

resident physicians gained experience in providing abortion care at outside institutions.[127] The discussion ended on the stark revelation that funds for graduate medical education and improved systems for away rotations are only the beginning of innovations needed to protect patient-centered care.

We are only just beginning to understand the impact of restrictions on reproductive rights as it pertains to trainees in medicine. We must continue to provide the time and space for our trainees to participate in these important conversations.

---

127 Accreditation Council for Graduate Medical Education. ACGME Program Requirements for Graduate Medical Education in Obstetrics and Gynecology Summary and Impact of Interim Requirement Revisions. Accreditation Council for Graduate Medical Education, 2022, https://www.acgme.org/globalassets/pfassets/reviewandcomment/220_obstetricsandgynecology_2022-06-24_impact.pdf

Looking Beyond the Uterus

Sarah Haynes, MD

Nothing instills more confidence in your patients than replying, "*uh, twelve weeks*" after they've asked how many years of experience you have as a doctor. With a mere twelve weeks under my belt, I make no diagnoses or decisions without the guidance of a more senior physician (thankfully).

My job as a first-year doctor is often to learn from the more experienced nurses and doctors who surround me. I've recently learned a valuable lesson about medicine's approach to women's health.

I started my evening shift, opened the list of patients waiting to be seen, and assigned myself first on the list. A young woman, around twenty weeks pregnant. I stepped into her room while my brain sorted through the collection of pregnancy-related conditions for potential diagnoses.

She was nauseous, febrile, with abdominal pain. I examined her tummy, thrown by the 20cm of growing uterus, I tried to localize her pain. Pain worse on the upper right side?

As all juniors do, I went to relay my assessment to the senior doctor in the emergency department that day. "*Call the obstetrics and gynaecology team.*"

An overworked and tired registrar answers the phone; *"so you've got a patient with a fever and abdominal pain who happens to be pregnant and currently has no red flag symptoms of a pregnancy-related emergency? Treat and examine this patient like any other nonpregnant patient who would present with these symptoms—call the surgeons."*

I assumed that this woman's pain was coming from her pregnant uterus and failed to consider other diagnoses. I shifted my thinking and considered what her collection of symptoms would make me concerned about in any non-pregnant patient. Gallstones?

Wrong again. She had appendicitis.

It hadn't even crossed my mind, and yet it's one of the first presentations of abdominal pain we are taught to identify in medical school. The most common identifying feature in appendicitis is pain in the right lower abdomen, and I missed that.

I've since learned appendicitis can present atypically in pregnant women. The right lower abdominal pain can often be felt higher in the abdomen, as the uterus grows and pushes the appendix higher.[128]

I was disappointed I couldn't look beyond the uterus to consider the whole patient. I had done what medicine has done to women for centuries; reduced their health to their reproductive organs. Something that is now coined as the "bikini approach" to women's health.

A quantitative analysis published in 2021 compared the research published in various women's health and general medical

---

128 Rebarber A, Jacob BP. "Acute Appendicitis in Pregnancy." UpToDate. 17 May 2022, https://www.uptodate.com/contents/acute-appendicitis-in-pregnancy

journals.[129] It found that 49% of women's health topics published in 2020 were on Reproductive Health. Furthermore, reproductive health was primarily focused on a woman's reproductive years. Women outside their reproductive years were significantly underrepresented in research. Only 2% of articles published were focused on menopause.[130]

After reproductive health, cancer was one of the most covered research topics. This was dominated by breast and cervical cancer with little focus on other significant cancers that disproportionately burden women, such as colorectal and lung cancer.[131]

Once upon a time, reproductive and maternal medicine was one of the greatest burdens on women's health, but maternal and infant mortality has improved throughout the twentieth century and the burden of disease has now shifted. The leading cause of death and disability for women is now noncommunicable diseases such as heart disease, respiratory disease, stroke, and cancers.[132] Then, there are the less common diseases that disproportionately affect women; women comprise 78% of people diagnosed with autoimmune diseases, around 66% of Alzheimer's disease, and are more likely to suffer from chronic pain.[133]

Women may live longer than men on average, but they live fewer healthier years than men. We know that sex and gender can affect the diagnosis and treatment of medical conditions. This has

---

129 Hallam, Laura et al. "Does Journal Content in the Field of Women's Health Represent Women's Burden of Disease? A Review of Publications in 2010 and 2020." *Journal of Women's Health*. vol. 31, no. 5, May 2022, pp. 611-619. doi: 10.1089/jwh.2021.0425

130 ibid.

131 ibid.

132 ibid.

133 Fairweather, DeLisa and Noel R. Rose. "Women and autoimmune diseases." *Emerging Infectious Diseases*. vol. 10, no. 11, Nov. 2004, pp. 2005-11. doi: 10.3201/eid1011.040367

been shown in the atypical presentation of heart attacks in women and how this ultimately leads to poorer outcomes.

While I am overjoyed to see more money and time spent on under-researched reproductive health conditions, such as endometriosis and polycystic ovarian syndrome, we must look beyond the uterus.

Medicine has spent centuries focusing on the 70kg white male and when it comes to the women, we've only been concerned about what lies beneath a bikini.

We must broaden the focus of what we consider to be "women's health" to adequately examine the role that sex and gender really play in the burden of disease.

Roe v. Wade and IVF/PGT

Rosemary B. Kirk, MD

The US Supreme Court's decision to revoke the constitutional right to an abortion has been widely and rightfully condemned. This decision will increase morbidity and mortality through unsafe abortions or the carrying of unwanted pregnancies, it infringes on the rights of pregnant people to make decisions about their bodies, and it will disproportionately affect individuals from marginalized communities. One consequence that may not be immediately obvious is the impact on people who have experienced infertility or genetic conditions.

When the *Roe v. Wade* ruling was made in 1973, research into assisted reproductive technology (ART) was in its infancy. The first successful *in vitro* fertilisation (IVF) birth occurred in 1978, and IVF now accounts for over 2% of US births.[134] A further technological gain alongside IVF has been pre-implantation genetic testing (PGT), first used in 1990,[135] and used in 27% of US ART cycles in

---

134 Centers for Disease Control and Prevention. "Assisted Reproductive Technology (ART)." Centers for Disease Control and Prevention, 16 Dec. 2021, https://www.cdc.gov/art/index.html.

135 Parikh, Firuza R. et al. "Preimplantation Genetic Testing: Its Evolution, Where Are We Today?" *Journal of Human Reproductive Sciences*. vol. 11, no. 4, Oct - Dec 2018, pp. 306-314. doi: 10.4103/jhrs.JHRS_132_18

2016.[136] In PGT, multiple embryos are produced through IVF, the embryos are screened for a pathogenic genetic variant or chromosomal abnormality, and only those embryos without abnormalities will be implanted. It is important to note that there are some ethical concerns associated with PGT, particularly when it is offered to screen for traits like embryo sex, or when polygenic-risk scores are used to judge lifetime disease risk or even intelligence (a poorly understood and ethically dubious science, and one that is not regulated in the US[137]). However, when PGT is used appropriately in patients who are carriers for life-threatening genetic conditions such as Huntington's disease, cystic fibrosis, or cancer-causing BRCA syndromes, it provides huge benefits. Patients who undergo PGT can not only prevent disease for their children but for all subsequent generations of their family. This reduces both individual suffering and the societal costs of long-term disease monitoring and treatment.

Despite the immense potential individual and societal benefits of IVF and PGT, they remain costly and relatively inaccessible in the US. There is no federal funding structure for IVF, and each IVF cycle costs an estimated $12,400-$24,000, with PGT serving as an additional expense. As of 2018, sixteen states had legislation mandating that insurers cover diagnosis and treatment of infertility, with only eight states specifically requiring that IVF be covered.[138]

136 Theobald, Rachel et al. "The status of preimplantation genetic testing in the UK and USA." *Human Reproduction.* vol. 35, no. 4, Apr. 2020, pp. 986-998. doi: 10.1093/humrep/deaa034

137 Goldberg, Carey. "Designer Babies: Parents Doing IVF Are Picking Embryos That Are 'Healthier'." Bloomberg, 17 Sept. 2021, https://www.bloomberg.com/news/articles/2021-09-17/picking-embryos-with-best-health-odds-sparks-new-dna-debate.

138 Peipert, Benjamin J. et al. "Impact of comprehensive state insurance mandates on in vitro fertilization utilization, embryo transfer practices, and outcomes in the United States." *American Journal of Obstetrics and Gynecology.* vol. 227, no. 1, Jul. 2022, pp. 64.e1-64.e8. doi: 10.1016/j.ajog.2022.03.003.

Consequently, most IVF/PGT is paid for out-of-pocket, and is inaccessible to many.

At a time when the US should be making efforts to increase accessibility to these reproductive technologies, the overturning of *Roe v. Wade* is a step backwards. IVF typically involves multiple embryos being produced to increase chances of success, and generally only one embryo is implanted to reduce the risks associated with multiple gestations. Remaining embryos may be discarded or stored with cryopreservation at great expense. The discarding of embryos is all but guaranteed when PGT is used, as some of the embryos produced will have life-threatening genetic variants. In states where abortion is banned from the time of fertilization, the discarding of embryos could become illegal, making it infeasible for clinics to continue to offer IVF and PGT.

Even beyond fertilization, the right to an abortion remains important throughout IVF pregnancies. Where IVF pregnancies result in a multiple gestation, either due to multiple embryos being transferred or due to embryos splitting, selective reduction may be used. This involves reducing the number of fetuses in order to reduce the risks of multiple gestation to the mother and remaining fetus(es). While this practice is declining as more IVF clinics perform only single-embryo transfer, it is still widely performed and will not be possible where abortion is illegal throughout pregnancy. Further, compared to other pregnancies, IVF pregnancies are at higher risk of complications that can pose risk to both mother and fetus including placental complications, need for blood transfusions or ICU admissions, and preterm births.[139] As such, abortion may be re-

---

139 Yanaihara, Atsushi et al. "Difference in the size of the placenta and umbilical cord between women with natural pregnancy and those with IVF pregnancy." *Journal of Assisted Reproduction and Genetics.* vol. 35, no. 3, Mar. 2018, pp. 431-434. doi: 10.1007/s10815-017-1084-2

quired to save the mother's life or to prevent the suffering of a fetus with major abnormalities by carrying it to term. In states where abortion is illegal with no exceptions, the decision to undertake a higher-risk IVF pregnancy will become significantly more complex and potentially dangerous.

Legalizing abortion increases women's rights to choose—to choose not to have children, but also *to have* children, or to choose to have children who are not at risk of genetic conditions. At a time when measures should be taken to increase access to IVF and PGT, the overturning of *Roe v. Wade* is a huge step backwards, not just for women's rights but for the fields of fertility and genetic medicine as a whole.

Thoughts on *Roe v Wade:* the Australian ED Trainee Perspective

Emily Williams, BM BS, BMedSci

I have looked after hundreds of patients, and none of them have the same story. People and disease cannot be forced into a trajectory or outcome that is desired or undesired—all we can do is provide modern, focused, and appropriate care and deal with what comes or doesn't.

I have looked after patients who have had a termination of pregnancy, those who are seeking a termination, those whose pregnancy has been unsuccessful despite how highly desired it was (both spontaneously conceived and via medical assistance), those who may still lose the pregnancy, those who are pregnant and miserable (some from physical symptoms, others from their social or environmental circumstances), those whose pregnancy is causing direct harm and risk to their health, those with foetal anomalies who may or will not survive after birth, and those who have uncomplicated, desired healthy pregnancies.

All of my patients, however, have been able to seek care freely with the knowledge that the law allows them to do so and that doctors will support their choices and target care to fit their specific needs.

Waking up to the overturning of *Roe v Wade* in the US was distressing, and I feel for my international colleagues and their patients in the wake of this.

The fundamental autonomy of both clinical practice and independent decision-making has been taken away from providers, placing a barrier to care in some locations and an extra burden to delivering this in others.

This will come at not only a high financial cost (no universal healthcare) but a massive societal one.

How is someone able to make an informed decision if they are too scared about punitive action? How do they then live with their choice?

How are they meant to find the money to pay for antenatal care, let alone financially provide for a child, when they couldn't afford to terminate the unplanned pregnancy that occurred because they had to choose between contraception and making rent?

How can doctors feel safe to provide targeted and appropriate care when the law isn't necessarily supporting them to do so?

How does it make a person feel when the state has declared that their life and the choices they make do not take precedence over a pregnancy that, before the gestation of viability, could not be sustained without them.

I am grateful for my rights, my training, and ability to care for all my patients in the best way I can and know how. I'm grateful I don't live and work in a polarized country where individuals are forgotten or decidedly ignored. I'm grateful that I can look after the scared, desperate, compromised, and vulnerable and truly help them to make informed decisions and that I am protected to do so.

In one of the richest nations in the world, I'm frightened that this ruling means others will have their decisions and rights questioned by those who do not live in their circumstances and have no concept of their lives, struggles, or trauma.

I thought that in the modern world, personal freedom was inherent—I guess in the case of the USA, perhaps not.

Why I Left, and Why It Matters

Joanna Bisgrove, MD, FAACP

*A year ago, I left a work situation that mimicked
what would happen if Roe fell. My story is a warning about how
the SCOTUS ruling on Dobbs v Jackson has forever changed
the US healthcare landscape for the worse.*

For fourteen years, I was a small-town, family physician in a state with a pre-Roe abortion ban. I took care of everyone who needed to be seen, but the heart and soul of my work centered on women and children. I took care of pregnant mothers, and I delivered and cared for their children. I also provided full reproductive health care, including counseling women with unplanned pregnancies on their options. That counseling, by the nature of my work, included the choice of an abortion.

It was this that put me at odds with my place of employment. Our group was bought out by a Catholic healthcare system about nine years ago. Over time, my increasing inability to effectively advocate for the needs of all of my patients frustrated me. Additionally, I could see the landscape of state politics shifting along with the changes in the makeup of the US Supreme Court. I could sense that the end of Roe was coming. So when a friend told me about a job opening at my medical school in a state where the right to abortion was protected, I jumped at the opportunity.

Why am I telling my story? Because as a physician and public health expert, it is my job to provide the best care for my patients based on science and the patient's personal needs. There is no place for anything else, yet outside interests keep trying to force their way in. For years, I fought it, but finally I couldn't anymore and I left. Now, what happened to me and my former colleagues threatens to play out in states across the country, and it could break the healthcare system.

Consider this: As family physicians, I and my partners in Wisconsin took care of well over 6,000 people in the region, with some traveling from over an hour away to see us. Since I've left, others have as well. There is now only one doctor and three physician assistants in the clinic and they cannot take care of everyone, leaving many to travel elsewhere to get care, even when they can't. It was agonizing leaving people I had developed such deep relationships with, and indeed I put off moving for years because I felt a duty to care for them. However, it got to the point where I knew if I stayed, I would have to choose between providing evidence-based care and the law. It was a choice I knew I could not make.

Now, multiply this by the thousands of doctors who live in states where abortion is now or about to be banned. A woman's ability to become pregnant impacts their care across medicine, from cancer care to rheumatology to infectious disease to everything in between, and all of us need the ability to help our patients make the best science and fact-based decisions for their own health. The vast majority of physicians will fight at first, but over time the fight will wear them down. Some will move, and some will leave medicine altogether. The result is that people lose their doctors.

Second, the Dobbs decision affects the future of medicine as well. A recent study found that, of study participants, 11% of physicians, physician trainees, or their partners previously had at least one abortion, no matter the specialty.[140] Additionally, 15% of medical student participants reported that either they or their partner previously had at least one abortion. Unintended pregnancy can delay and potentially derail years of expensive medical training. It's a chance many young physicians and physician trainees cannot afford to take. They will, therefore, be less likely to apply to medical school, apply for residency, or take a job in a state where abortion is banned. As a result, the gaps in access to care for all patients in states where abortion is banned will become significant.

Third, male physicians are affected. As noted above, the study also cited partners of physicians who had abortions. Additionally, the most recent available data on couples matching showed that over 1,000 couples participated in the residency couples matching process in 2019, and that number grows every year.[141] That is a not insignificant number of couples who could now also be looking to avoid states where abortion is banned.

To be sure, much of what I am saying is hypothetical. I cannot possibly know what is happening in the minds of doctors in states

---

140 Levy, Morgan S. et al. "Abortion Among Physicians." *Obstetrics and Gynecology.* vol. 139, no. 5, May 2022, pp. 910-912. doi: 10.1097/AOG.0000000000004724
141 Murphy, Brendan. "Perfecting it as a pair: The do's and don'ts of the Couples Match." American Medial Association, Dec. 2019, https://www.ama-assn.org/ medical-students/preparing-residency/perfecting-it-pair-do-s-and-don-ts-couples-match#:~:text=Still%2C%20if%20you%27re%20attempting,Sacotte%20said.

where abortion is or will be banned. But I can say this: in my previous job, I am, by far, not the only one who has left. Many of us who did disagreed with the overriding principles espoused by our parent organization. Additionally, the number of physicians who have left, combined with the difficulty in replacing us during a nationwide shortage of doctors, means that the care the organization can provide is impacted. What's happened in my old place of employment is now a very real scenario for healthcare across the country.

We are entering uncharted waters as a country, and a handful of supreme court justices who have no understanding of healthcare just made a decision that impacts the entirety of the profession and the people we serve. People from all walks of life will be affected by this decision, not just women who seek an abortion and related services. The story I have told is just one facet of what is to come, but it is one which cannot be ignored.

Conclusion:
Sincerely, Cassandra
and Bruno

Avital O'Glasser, MD, FACP, SFHM, DFPM

Dear friends, family, colleagues, and concerned(ish) public:

It's likely very difficult for you to have imagined what this month, January 2023, would have been like if you had been asked to predict it three years ago. Me? Cassandra? Aw heck, I could have told you what to expect—but if you had asked, or even listened, odds were you would not have been able to believe me. (I shake my fist at you, Apollo, for that damn curse of seeing the future but never being believed!) At least my name finally crept into the collective vernacular with people saying they *feel* like me or should get their names changed to "Cassandra." Meanwhile, Bruno over here? Heck, you didn't even know he existed until 2021. (That, and the fact that *we don't talk about Bruno*.)

I will say, though, with the help of a global pop-culture phenomenon, and with some people's return to the Classics (I guess there's only so much a person can stream online while they waited for the third season of Ted Lasso...), it is really nice to have some more name—and brand—recognition.

One of our most validating experiences in the last year came when the Merriam Webster (MW) dictionary announced "gaslighting" as the 2022 word of the year (WOTY).[142] MW owns their decision in the most mic-drop way possible: "It is totally a real word, and not something we made up just to mess with you."[143] Wait—did MW just say they aren't gaslighting us about the meaning of the word "gaslighting?"

The MW word of the year doesn't need to be a brand-new word. "Gaslighting" originates from the 1938 play "Gas Light" that... you guessed it...demonstrated that concept as a core plot element. The choice is driven by the frequency at which certain words are looked up in the dictionary in the past year. "Gaslighting" saw a 1740% increase.[144] The 2021 WOTY was "vaccine"; in 2020 it was "pandemic." I'm seeing a theme emerge...maybe the 2023 word will be "I'm taking public health experts and epidemiologists seriously." Oh wait...that's a phrase, not a word... And damn it, "I told you so" is a phrase, too! Bruno is whispering to me that he's putting his money on "Weltschmerz," the feeling of "world weariness" or the feeling you get "when your expectations of the world fall disappointingly short."[145]

Bruno and I might seem cool and aloof, throwing shade at

142 "Word of the Year 2022." Merriam-Webster, 2022, https://www.merriam-webster.com/words-at-play/word-of-the-year.
143 Merriam-Webster [@MerriamWebster]. "Some Things You Should Know about 'Gaslighting': It Had a 1740% Increase in Lookups for the Past Year.- It Comes from the Title of a 1938 Play (and the Movie Based on That Play).- It Is Totally a Real Word, and Not Something We Made up Just to Mess with You." Twitter, 28 Nov. 2022, https://twitter.com/MerriamWebster/status/1597232594344501248?s=20&t=QkHeCxnXGL24PVU601aglw.
144 Merriam-Webster [@MerriamWebster]. "Some Things You Should Know about 'Gaslighting': It Had a 1740% Increase in Lookups for the Past Year.- It Comes from the Title of a 1938 Play (and the Movie Based on That Play).- It Is Totally a Real Word, and Not Something We Made up Just to Mess with You." Twitter, 28 Nov. 2022, https://twitter.com/MerriamWebster/status/1597232594344501248?s=20&t=QkHeCxnXGL24PVU601aglw.
145 Lewis, Benny. "13 Badass German Words We Really Need in English." Fluentin3months. https://www.fluentin3months.com/badass-german-words/

the states of denial paraded around as blissful ignorance, wishful thinking, or unrealistic optimism. Like Katie Porter,[146] it might appear that we don't give a F*...but that is just our psychological defense mechanism. We really do care, we really do give a F*...but we are truly running out of F*'s left to give. So here we are, with our siblings in advocacy, desperately trying to spread the messages that are either ignored or that don't want to be talked about.

No, the pandemic isn't over.

Yes, COVID is still here.

No, the COVID vaccine is not killing thousands of people.

Yes, we DO know how to stop COVID's spread.

No, healthcare worker morale is not getting any better.

Yes, hospitals are over capacity and the healthcare system is crumbling.

No, you cannot avoid RSV and the flu just by wishful thinking.

Yes, the third season of Ted Lasso is long overdue (we believe everyone DOES agree on that one...go figure...).

Against the flood of misinformation, disinformation, and disbelief, we know some of you are listening, standing up, and speaking out. On your behalf, I'm going to channel Bruno's eloquent niece: "Gimme the truth and the whole truth, Bruno."

Bruno and I have built the bonds of an unlikely friendship through shared experience and mutual understanding over the past year. It has made our necessary missions a bit less isolating. A lone duck became a pair . . . so hey Lin-Manuel, ya gonna write us a new partner in crime this year, a new comrade in arms, a third musketeer? We'll believe it when we see it.

Sincerely,

Cassandra and Bruno

---

146 Carter, Simone. " Katie Porter Goes Viral for Reading This Book During Chaotic Speaker Fight." *Newsweek*. January 7, 2023. https://www.newsweek.com/katie-porter-goes-viral-reading-this-book-during-chaotic-speaker-fight-1772069

Epilogue: About a Daughter Who Wants to Become a Doctor

Anika Tulsi Kumar (Age 9)

Hi, my name is Anika, the daughter of the amazing doctor mom, Dr. Shikha Jain, and I will tell you she is a *great* doctor mom. I am a future doctor. You might be wondering, what does it feel like to have a doctor-mom and doctor family? Take my advice, having a doctor family is a blast, especially when your mom and dad are doctors.

My mom really inspired me to become a doctor, teacher, scientist, mom, all these amazing jobs, because she is a very kind person who wants to change the world. Dr. Jain spends the most time with me, my doctor dad known as Dr. Kumar and my two brothers, and gets her work done too! Dr. Jain can single task, and she can multitask. The most amazing part about her is that she's kind to others even if they are not kind to her.

In my opinion, the doctors in my family take things and make them better. For example, my mom is working on improving women's rights because women deserve to be heard. It's also nice to have people at home who can help you when you are sick, or you get hurt. I also love to see how the doctors and nurses in my family help others when they are sick. In our family, my mom is a doctor (as you all know), my dad is a doctor, my grandpa is a surgeon, my dad's mom is a nurse, and my uncle and auntie in India are dentists.

When I visited India, where much of my extended family lives, I saw a lot of homeless and sick people and felt even more the need to be a doctor to help as many people as I can.

I feel so lucky to have so many people who love me and can also take care of me when I am sick or hurt. My doctor mom and dad also help other family and friends when they get sick, and it makes me feel good that they can help so many people.

When I was younger, I thought I would become a flower... a beautiful sunflower when I grew up. Now I want to be like my mom, but we'll see what happens when I'm older!

If you want to become a doctor, you have to be a lot of things. First, you have to be responsible. Second, you *have* to be patient with your patients. (That was a joke if nobody noticed, but if you want to become a doctor you still have to be patient with your patient.) Third, you have to be good at communicating scary and difficult things to all sorts of people. And if someone speaks a different language, it helps if you know more than one language (not all of them though). Fourth, one thing my mom has taught me is that you need to stand up for what's right, no matter how hard it may be.

Additional Perspective From Anika's Mom

Shikha Jain, MD, FACP

When I informed my nine-year-old daughter that we would be curating a collection of works by individuals of all genders on the subject of women in medicine, her initial request was, "Can I write something for the book?"

We all lead multifaceted lives, wearing numerous hats and becoming experts at code-switching in our daily routines. Doctor, mother, wife, daughter, sister, caregiver, partner—our roles fluctuate from day to day, sometimes even from minute to minute. We transition from delivering life-altering news to a patient's family to shuttling kids between sports and extracurricular activities. We coordinate doctors' appointments for aging parents while grappling with the challenges of infertility, pregnancy, or miscarriages, and then find ourselves performing heart transplants in the operating room. As the saying goes, we are expected to work as if we don't have families and care for our families as if we don't have jobs. Although my children understand that I inhabit multiple spaces, it doesn't make it any less difficult to leave them in the morning or miss a recital or soccer game due to my other responsibilities.

I launched the Women in Medicine Summit shortly after delivering my twin boys. I can still vividly recall the moment when the concept of the programming and its intent came to me. Returning from maternity leave, I felt a pressing need to address the challenges that women in medicine encounter on a daily basis. For years, I attributed my personal failures and difficulties to an inherent problem with myself—my intelligence, skills, and abilities. I couldn't recognize toxic environments or overt harassment because I had been conditioned to believe that this was simply the way things were. It wasn't until I momentarily stepped out of that environment and began listening to other women's stories that I realized many of us shared similar experiences. The problem wasn't us; it was the system.

Despite the privilege of having an incredibly supportive family while growing up, I completely overlooked the implicit discrimination and harassment that permeated my life as a woman in medicine. I had not only normalized it, but I had unquestioningly accepted it. As I spoke with more women, I realized the urgent need to not only bring greater attention to this issue but to also empower others to identify such problems in real-time and address them. My aim was to empower individuals of all genders to critically examine our systems and collaborate in disrupting them to bring about positive change.

It is essential not only to empower women but also to encourage allies to step up and rectify the wrongs. We must emphasize the impact of these pervasive inequities on individuals with intersectional identities, such as women of color. And then, we must provide opportunities for these individuals to drive change—leadership positions, awards, chances to shine on national and international platforms. Thus, the Women in Medicine Summit was born. Fast forward through a pandemic, during which women in medicine demonstrated remarkable resilience and leadership beyond what should have been expected, and witnessed the exodus of brilliant women from healthcare due to unfavorable working conditions, harassment, a loss of autonomy, and burnout—I felt compelled to do more.

The Women in Medicine Summit, and subsequently the Women in Medicine™ nonprofit, emerged from the need to fix the system. We aimed to empower women and their allies while simultaneously providing opportunities, fostering networks, and amplifying the persisting challenges in healthcare to achieve equity for healthcare workers. Our goal has always been to work towards real solutions.

I am immensely grateful for all the phenomenal individuals who have contributed to our growth as a powerful community. I am humbled by those who attend the conference and share their stories. I extend my thanks to all those who have placed their trust in me, this organization, and the Summit to create a space where everyone has the opportunity to share their vulnerabilities, uplift others, and rise together.

Becoming a doctor has been my lifelong aspiration, but I never imagined my career would lead me down this path. I am forever grateful for the opportunity to meet and engage with countless amazing individuals through this platform and these networks. This organization and conference have truly transformed my life. Whatever the future holds for Women in Medicine™ and the Women in Medicine Summit, I am cautiously optimistic that together, we can drive change. Because at the end of the day, we are, and will always be, stronger together.

Acknowledgments

This book—this powerful anthropology of empowered voices—is the result of the energy and investments of many people. This work would not exist without the creative energies of the more than seventy authors themselves. We thank them for sharing their voice and vulnerability with us—first by submitting their pieces to the WIMS Blog and then again when giving their permission to share in this book. When we launched the WIMS Blog in July 2021, we had no idea how wide and loud the beautiful music of these voices would be—and here we are now, sharing this symphonic accomplishment.

Thank you to our families and loved ones—especially our spouses and our children who champion, cheer, and energize our work, as well as our parents, who never said we "couldn't" because we were girls. Thank you to the friends, colleagues, peers, mentors, sponsors, and allies who lift us up during our efforts to lift others. This includes our colleagues Drs. Vineet Arora, Mark Shapiro, and Charlie Wray in the Advancing Vitae and Novel Contributions for Everyone (ADVANCE) group and all those challenging norms in medicine and academia to honor and recognize the inherent worth and impact of nontraditional scholarship such as the WIMS Blog.

Thank you to Women in Medicine™ (WIM) and the Women in Medicine Summit (WIMS)—and the faculty leads, students, and advisors who make these organizations excel at fulfilling their missions. We are thankful for their direct support of the WIMS Blog and this book as well as their broader, overarching support for gender equity and allyship in medicine. Drs. Eve Bloomgarden, Tricia Pendergrast, Neelum Aggarwal, Parul Barry, Ananya Gangopadhyaya, Julie Oyler, and Anjana Pillai have been with WIMS since the beginning and without their efforts and continued support, none of this would have been possible. And to Polly Rossi and the Meeting Achievements team who have helped to support and grow WIM and WIMS since their inception, as well as Drs. Arghavan Salles and Annabelle Volgman—thank you for your continued support and guidance.

Another thanks goes to the team at Healio's Women in Oncology series, especially Sasha Todak and Jennifer Southall, for their collaboration with us to continue to elevate women's voices in medicine. In February 2022, our blogs started collaborating and cross-posting blog pieces. Nearly a dozen posts that originally appeared on the Healio Women in Oncology blog are now included in this book, and we thank the authors and Healio for their permission to be included here.

And finally, our most gracious thanks to our support team who provided the most hands-on support to complete this book— Leeana Penumalee, University of Chicago Pritzker School of Medicine student who was instrumental with her editing and manuscript preparation; Dr. Davy Ran who gifted us with their magnificent cover art in addition to their two essays; Dr. Kimberly Manning who honored us with her invited preface; and Idie Benjamin whose financial support helped us cross the finish line.

Author Index

You can find individual authors' pieces on the following pages.

About the Authors

Dr. Avital O'Glasser is a professor of medicine and hospitalist at Oregon Health & Science University (OHSU). She holds dual appointments in the Division of Hospital Medicine and the Department of Anesthesiology and Perioperative Medicine at OHSU. Driven by her commitment to comprehensive, patient-centered, interdisciplinary patient-centered care, she is the Medical Director of OHSU's Preoperative Medicine Clinic. Dr. O'Glasser is a fervent advocate for exploring the intersection of medicine and nontraditional scholarship. She explores how social media can effectively contribute to the field of medicine and foster collaboration and knowledge dissemination among healthcare professionals. In her pursuit of promoting gender equity and other diversity, equity, and inclusion (DEI) initiatives, Dr. O'Glasser advocates for recognition of novel contributions including digital scholarship and advocacy. She inspires and empowers fellow healthcare professionals to embrace new avenues of impact and strive for a more equitable and inclusive future in medicine. Her energies and efforts have been honored with institutional, regional, and national awards including the American College of Physician's Walter McDonald Early Career Physician award.

Dr. Shikha Jain is a distinguished board-certified hematology and oncology physician and unwavering advocate for advancing medicine and empowering women. As a tenured associate professor at the University of Illinois Cancer Center, she leaves a transformative impact through groundbreaking research, advocacy efforts, and compassionate clinical care. As Director of Communications, Dr. Jain bridges the gap between medical knowledge and public understanding, championing digital technologies for enhanced patient care and countering misinformation through media channels. Passionate about empowering women in medicine and positively disrupting the healthcare system, she is Founder and President of the nonprofit Women in Medicine™ and the Women in Medicine Summit™, fostering inclusivity within the medical community. As CEO and Co-Founder of IMPACT, Dr. Jain amplifies the voices of healthcare professionals, advocating for actionable change. Her dedication earned recognition as one of Medscape's 25 Rising Stars and Modern Healthcare's Top 25 Emerging Leaders. A respected authority, Dr. Jain's insightful contributions shed light on crucial healthcare topics. Captivating keynote speeches and groundbreaking work position her at the forefront of medical innovation.

Made in United States
North Haven, CT
14 September 2023

41552006R00183